HIIT

Learn How and Why Hiit Shreds Fat and How to
Implement Starting Today!

(Hiit Bicycle Training Guide Harness the Power of
High Intensity)

Michael Flynn

Published by Harry Barnes

Michael Flynn

HIIT: Learn How and Why Hiit Shreds Fat and How to Implement Starting Today! (Hiit Bicycle Training Guide Harness the Power of High Intensity)

ISBN 978-1-77485-135-7

Legal & Disclaimer

The information contained in this book is not designed to replace or take the place of any form of medicine or professional medical advice. The information in this book has been provided for educational and entertainment purposes only.

The information contained in this book has been compiled from sources deemed reliable, and it is accurate to the best of the Author's knowledge; however, the Author cannot guarantee its accuracy and validity and cannot be held liable for any errors or omissions. Changes are periodically made to this book. You must consult your doctor or get professional medical advice before using any of the suggested remedies, techniques, or information in this book.

Upon using the information contained in this book, you agree to hold harmless the Author from and against any damages, costs, and expenses, including any legal fees potentially resulting from the application of any of the information provided by this guide. This disclaimer applies to any damages or injury caused by the use and application, whether directly or indirectly, of any advice or information presented, whether for breach of contract, tort, negligence, personal injury, criminal intent, or under any other cause of action.

You agree to accept all risks of using the information presented inside this book. You need to consult a professional medical practitioner in order to ensure you are both able and healthy enough to participate in this program.

Table of Contents

Introduction

One of the problems with exercise is that it can take a long time to get the results you're looking for. High intensity interval training (HIIT) is one of the most effective methods of exercise. It is now the top workout for many professional athletes who need to get fit fast. In this guide, you'll learn how you can gain massive fitness results without spending hours at the gym.

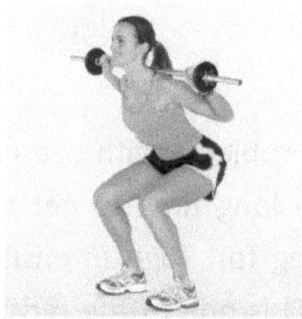

We all realize the importance of regular exercise, not only for the overall health benefits, but also to gain energy, lose weight and gain strength. The problem is, if we have to invest a lot of money or time on equipment gym memberships, or coaching, it can be easy to not make exercise a priority.

One of the most powerful things about HIIT is that it really fits into our busy lifestyle and, in many cases, we can do it at home with some basic equipment. This is one workout method that does not need a lot of fancy equipment or massive amounts of time to see results.

The basic premise of HIIT is to engage small intervals of exercise that is of high intensity. In between, moderate or low levels of exertion are being used. By alternating between very hard, but brief, exercise duration, and then a less intense one, the metabolism keeps working in the heart rate stays up long after the session is finished.

What's great about HI IT is that you are building strength and also improving your endurance levels.

This guide covers everything you need to get started with an effective HIIT program. You'll learn the benefits, how to get started, and how to effectively work out.

Chapter 1: Will Hiit Work For Me?

Short answer, heck yea, long answer keep reading! You see the reason HIIT works for anyone and everyone is because you can totally individualize the workout. It does not matter if you're just a beginner or an avid marathon runner HIIT will work for you. Of course if I'm just beginning my exercise journey the way I program and do a HIIT workout to start with will be vastly different from someone who's an ultra marathon runners (marathoners who run 100 miles in a single race and sometimes more, crazy right?) You don't even have to be a marathoner to get HIIT to work for you, HIIT works great for the avid powerlifter who wants to lean down, the mom that doesn't have the time to go to the gym, and at home workout enthusiasts. Regardless what background you have HIIT will work for you to lean down and tone up and here's how.

You see after we do a HIIT workout it causes what we call "Excess Post-Exercise Oxygen Consumption" or EPOC for short, I know I know lots of acronyms in this but you'll catch on quick! I think I can, I think I can! Right? Anyways what EPOC means is that after exercise our body needs more oxygen to catch up after all the work we did! Because of this our body starts collecting more oxygen. This oxygen is then used to help rebuild our body after we broke it down a little bit which causes a caloric burn. About 5 calories are burned to one liter of oxygen ingestion. Not only that but HIIT has been proven to increase the effects of EPOC in less time over other forms of exercise like stable state cardio. Stable state cardio being an exercise like walking, jogging, or cycling for an extended period of time.

Not only does HIIT cause EPOC but because of the high intensity nature of the workout it increases our levels of HGH a.k.a. Human growth hormone! This leads to more defined muscles that are leaner and stronger. This happens because with HIIT our muscles develop microtears which when we supply our muscles with the right foods causes them to heal and come back stronger, and yes these microtears are what causes same day muscles tiredness and the typical soreness we have the next day. Wanna know what's so great about growing our muscles? We get even more calorie burn! Fat in our body just sits there but because our muscles always need fuel to move our body even when we are sitting muscles still burn calories. This is the surprising truth about getting a lean muscular body, we actually should be wanting to gain some muscle tone! But don't worry without some serious resistance training this muscle growth won't cause bulkiness but that lean, and toned look that I'm sure you're after, and even if you're not and want to be bigger add in some weightlifting! *Cough* But this books about not using a gym *cough* so let's move on!

HIIT will also work for you if you are looking to save time! Everyone knows that you should get in 30 minutes of cardio a couple times a week but how boring is that? Okay, okay, I'm a little biased but even if you truly do enjoy running what if you're on a time crunch and only have 15 minutes to get some running in? Hard to hit your weight loss goals when you have to cut out half your workout! But guess what you can cut down on your workout time significantly with HIIT! Imagine 10 minutes of your day and you'll burn more calories than 30 minutes of jogging! How is that not for everyone.

Another great benefit of HIIT is you will see results even if you don't want to change your nutrition. Now I'm not recommending this route at all but I'm not going to twist your arm to convince you otherwise, some of my clients only work with me for my exercise programming and one such example is one of my clients named Beth. Beth was well into her 40's but adding two HIIT sessions a week definitely changed her body, and her life. She became leaner and in six weeks, without any nutritional changes she lost around 5% of her body fat! Granted she just began her exercise journey (change happens a little bit quicker when we're new since our body hasn't adapted to working out yet) but that's a fantastic result. This result is possible, all you need to do is put in the work!

Chapter 2: How To Use Hiit?

To start your HIIT journey you simply need to pick one exercise you are happy with one you can perform at varying levels of intensity. Jogging/running is the most cost effective and more commonly used in the first trial with HIIT.

You'll need a stop watch and a plan.

Set your stop watch running and for the first 45 seconds you'll just be jogging or walking, anything that you can sustain easily for 10 minutes or so, from a ranking score of 1 to 10, 1 being no effort at all and 10 being using as much effort as physically possible you should be at about 4. As soon as the stop watch gets to 45 seconds to crank the intensity up to 10, don't worry this is only going to last for 15 seconds so get it as much as you can and you'll feel the benefits at the end.

Repeat this low intensity high intensity cycle ten times, that gives you a super effective workout in 10 minutes and benefits that will last for up to 2 days, just in time for you to repeat the same workout again and ramp up your metabolism.

To perform HIIT we need a specific exercise to use to demonstrate the format, I have chosen jogging and running because anyone can do it with a small amount of equipment and the financial cost can be zero.

Once you've completed a respectable warm up and I'm not going to teach you to suck eggs but a sufficient warm up should leave you feeling warm (surprise) and slightly clammy, it should also be specific to the type of activity to be undertaken so in it's simplest terms warming up for a run would be achieved by walking, jogging and dynamically stretching the muscles involved in that movement.

I would always recommend that you start of with a low intensity period just so your body and mind has time to adapt to the

required stresses being forced upon it. The timings are up to you but in my opinion if this is your first time I would treat with caution until you are more aware of your limitation.

Your workout should look like this:

Jog/walk

45 seconds

Run/sprint

15 seconds

Jog/walk

45 seconds

Run/sprint

15 seconds

Jog/walk

45 seconds

Run/sprint

15 seconds

Jog/walk

45 seconds

Run/sprint

15 seconds

Jog/walk

45 seconds

Run/sprint

15 seconds

Jog/walk

45 seconds

Run/sprint

15 seconds

Jog/walk

45 seconds

Run/sprint

15 seconds

Jog/walk

45 seconds

Run/sprint

15 seconds

Jog/walk

45 seconds

Run/sprint

15 seconds

Jog/walk

45 seconds

Run/sprint

15 seconds

You'll notice that you are never completely resting, so even in the Low Intensity periods were you are getting your breath back your body is still having to metabolise energy to induce movement, just at a much slower pace. This twinned with the short bursts of maximum effort are the fundamental keys to creating rapid fat loss, skimp on the 100% effort and you are only cheating yourself.

This workout from start to finish will last 10 minutes, this is about 0.069% of your day, now I don't care if you are a neuroscientist or the Prime Minister of England you will have time to complete this workout so using the 'I don't have time' excuse is no longer valid.

Once you've used this workout a number of times a week and have got used to the intensity levels required you can do one of four things to build on the intensity.

1. Increase the period working at HI

2. Decrease the period working at LI

3. Add another set making the work out 3 min 20 sec long

4. Change the exercise to something more intense

It looks like a lot but it will only last for 10 minutes, it's going to be uncomfortable but again it's only going to last 10 minutes.

Try using this app 'gymboss' it's super easy to use and allows you to programme in as many timings as you need.

How to set goals so you guarantee success

Ok so now we established the method of exercise to be used to achieve your goals and we know that it is possibly the most effective way to lose fat through exercise we need to talk about the second most important and effective step of achieving success........setting your goals.

1. Step one is deciding what your goal actually looks like and putting it in writing, the power of writing down a specific goal is incredibly powerful not only because you have decided exactly what your goals

is but by writing down on paper solidifies that goal and purpose in your mind.

You Must Be Specific, saying you want to lose weight and get in shape is not enough, you must define a weight loss amount and actual figure in pounds or kilograms or if your

goal is to fit into a dress or pair of jeans write it down make sure its something quantifiable, something you can measure and actual recognise when you achieve it.

2. Pure Belief

Without belief in yourself you will not achieve your goal and continue when things get tough and you can't be bothered, you inner voice will tell you you are not good enough, you don't have what it takes and whats the point anyway. Self-belief is possibly the biggest reason anybody doesn't achieve something they have set out to accomplish. You can do this and should constantly tell yourself, it's like Henry Ford said

'If you believe you can or believe you can't, in both cases you're probably right'. If somebody else has achieved something you want to achieve then there is no reason why you can't achieve that goal as well.

You Can Do It!

3. Write a plan and anticipate barriers

Write down your plan for achieving your goal on paper, the exercises and the timings, leave nothing to chance know without any doubt what it is you're going to have to do to reach your goal, so when it comes to the moment of starting to exercise you know exactly what is expected of you. As well as this anticipate possible barriers to this exercise routine and what you will if they happen for example you want to exercise when you get home from work before your evening meal but you could get caught in traffic and take longer to get home than expected, what will you do? Or you plan to skip at different intensity's but the dog eats the skipping rope, what will you do? Having a plan B is essential if you are planning for success, let nothing get in your way.

4. Measure

If your goal is to drop 5 inches from your waist, measure your waist, if you want to drop 5% body fat measure your body fat. Keep track of your progress, it's one of the most motivating tricks actually seeing what you've achieved and without it your mind will try and trick you into thinking you've done nothing especially when you're feeling low so don't leave it to chance write those stats down and congratulate yourself every time you get a step closer to your goal.

5. Review and learn

Review your stats every week, be honest and evaluate how well you've done this week, could you have pushed harder if so why and why didn't you. Did you miss any sessions, if so why and more importantly what can you do to make you don't miss more sessions in the future. Every week you should be evolving into a more effective and efficient individual so that in 2 months nothing gets in your way and nothing stops you from smashing every goal you set yourself.

Simply follow these 5 steps to setting and achieving your

HIIT goals and you will easily double your chances of success and being a happier person, you deserve it and yes you can do it!

The top 5 reasons why you don't exercise and what you can do to smash them to pieces

There are literally hundreds of reasons why you shouldn't exercise, if you're left to think about and procrastination sets in you can easily dream up many barriers and 'other things' you would rather be up to what you need to do is fully decide why you want to exercise and more importantly what benefits you're going to receive from being slimmer, healthier and happier.

The number one reason you don't exercise is because you don't have time. You have time to watch T.V, check Facebook, look at websites and even do chores but for some reason you don't have time to exercise.

This is a myth and you need to rule your mind on this one set 20 minutes out of your day to exercise and when you get to that time discipline yourself to know you do have time because you have scheduled it into your day. Everyone can find 20 minutes in their day to exercise if you sit down and really schedule it in after all you don't need to travel to a gym you do HIIT, it is in your home or at most it is outside your front door.

The number two reason you don't exercise is you're too tired.

Guess what, scientific research shows that if you exercise it gives you energy makes you feel revitalised and puts a spring in your step. Try it once and if you feel more tired after HIIT than when you started I will refund the price of this ebook, the reason I make this offer is because I'm so confident it won't happen.

To set a test, before you exercise score yourself on how tired you feel between 1 and 10, 1 being dead on your feet and 10 being super charged on caffeine and once you've finished score yourself again between 1 and 10. I guarantee your second score will be higher than your first score.

The number three reason you don't exercise is its too boring.

HIIT is so dynamic and versatile you can literally adapt any physical activity can be used in the HIIT template, so this is boring you only have yourself to blame. Use your imagination and find something that excites you, hell you can even use sex.

The number four reason you don't exercise is it's too expensive.

HIIT is free, the app I have recommended is free, you don't need any equipment if you're running and jogging, you can make it as expensive or as cost effective as you like so you will all ways have enough money to exercise.

The number five reason and the biggest of barriers to exercise is you tell yourself you've tried it before and you haven't been able to make it work, **you don't believe you can see it through because maybe you haven't done it before.**

Just start, even in a small way it doesn't matter your aim is to be better than you were before, stop comparing yourself to someone else other people have their only journey and their own troubles that is none of your business as long as you are consistently trying you will achieve your goal, failure is not possible if you never give up and if you never give up you will at some point succeed.

You must tell yourself and believe that this time is different, this time you have HIIT and it will work.

Chapter 3: Is Hiit Training For You

To be honest, almost any individual can give HIIT a go, as long as you are up for the intensity of training, especially in the beginning. This is not to say that it gets easier with time but, the hardest part of any training regimen or sport has always been the beginning...getting your body used to working large groups of muscles at a time and getting accustomed to raised heart and breathing rate levels is not something many people are cut out for.

If you are looking for a new, challenging training method then, HIIT is for you. If you are a beginner or have recently recovered from an injury, then HIIT is still a viable option for you, so long as you take it one step at a time and do not push yourself to hard. Although HIIT training can be done by almost anyone, it is important to ensure that you are capable of doing at 15 to 20 minutes of uninterrupted exercise without any problems, before you jump into HIIT full force. If your body cannot withstand basic exercise, it is probably best to consult with a medical professional or certified fitness expert before attempting any strenuous activity or, you could just avoid HIIT training altogether. At the end of the day, fitness training methods should be about improving and building your body, not exerting and tearing it down.

The American College of Sports Medicine cites sedentary lifestyles along with other factors just as genetics, high cholesterol levels, smoking, obesity and many other issues as contributing factors to the increase in your chances of developing serious health problems, should you undertake high intensity workout methods. They advise checking and consulting with your doctor before taking up HIIT training.

Now that we have established that who can do HIIT training and who should take caution, we should take a closer look at some of the health benefits this progressive training method has to offer.

Health Benefits

As I mentioned before, high intensity interval training is quite popular in the world of fitness and this can be boiled down to its unique approach to training that combines maximum effort with shorter training time as well as its many health benefits. HIIT training provides a good boost to your metabolism in addition to burning a lot of calories in a fairly short time. Some other health benefits of HIIT include:

Building endurance

High intensity interval training changes your muscles' cellular structure thus, allowing you to raise your endurance levels during any form of exercise. A study was conducted and posted in the Journal of Physiology, where people undertook HIIT training for 8 weeks. The results revealed an increase (double) in the amount of time they were able to cycle while maintaining the exact same pace.

Faster burning of calories

If you are looking for a training method that burns fat and calories at a fast rate and in a short time frame then HIIT might be the perfect option for you. Research has revealed that less than 20 minutes of HIIT training burns a greater number of calories compared to hour long treadmill workouts. The East Tennessee State University conducted a study in 2001 and found that when trainees stuck to an 8 week high intensity interval training program, their body fat percentage dropped by 2% as opposed to those who were following a steadier workout program who experienced no change in their body fat percentage at all. They also found that trainees of HIIT burnt as much as 100 calories more each day during the full day of each workout. Another study carried out in 2007, showed that females who had undertaken high intensity interval training over a period of two weeks had an increase in fat oxidation of up to 30% and were able to lose weight a lot faster that women who were doing regular, steadier cardio exercises.

Energy is used more effectively

High intensity interval training teaches your body to use energy more effectively through a system of maximum effort coupled with short recovery periods. In addition to this, toxic waste is removed from the muscles while you are recovering. You also breathe more effectively when you alternate between workouts.

Saves time

Regular workouts tend to be time consuming and lengthy and as such, not everyone is excited to complete a full workout. In addition to this, spending prolonged periods of time on a treadmill, for example, could be detrimental to your joints and overall health and in many cases, the results are not as quick and effective as those of high intensity interval training. It is possible to tailor HIIT to your experience and limit and you are still guaranteed fat burning benefits even if your workout is as short as 15 minutes about two to three times per week. This can help you get your desired results in a shorter amount of time while saving your joints and overall health from the pressures of continuous exposure to long and repetitive workouts.

Better metabolism

The American College of Sports and Medicine has credited HIIT with helping people consume a greater amount of oxygen compared to non-interval training methods. This in turn, aids the body's metabolism by increasing it to higher rates during the 90-144 minute period after an interval training session. This increase in metabolism helps the body burn a greater number of calories at a much faster rate.

Continued fat and calorie burning hours after training

Higher intensity training methods boost the body's ability to repair itself after workouts. Within a day after finishing an HIIT session, your body will still be burning fat and calories, something steadier paced workouts may not offer.

HIIT training requires little to no equipment

One of the benefits that high intensity interval training offers is affordability and this can be credit to its requirement of little to no equipment when training. With a bit of open space and your body weight, you can engage in intense, calorie burning workouts and enjoy amazing results at a very low cost. That is not say that you cannot add weights or other equipment to your training regimen but, you really do not have to. In some cases, equipment such as weights could actually slow you down and interrupt the intensity of your workout.

Shreds fat instead of muscle

Regular cardio exercises have often been reported to result in loss of valuable muscle mass. With high intensity interval training, however, that is not a concern as it pairs weight (body) training with other high intensity cardio exercises to ensure that muscle is preserved while excess fat is being trimmed. One particular review found that when over 400 individuals who were classified as obese or overweight undertook HIIT and moderate exercise, both were effective at reducing the circumference of the waistline as well as reducing body fat. Another study found that undertaking high intensity interval training for 20 minutes/session for about 3 times a week resulted in a weight loss of up to 4+ pounds in a space of just twelve weeks...all this without having paired up the regimen with the necessary diet. The fat that causes and promotes disease in the body (usually located around the vital organs) was also reduced by up to 17 per cent. Many other studies have been successfully conducted and further proved that high intensity interval training was effective for reducing the body's fat levels. As mentioned before, this is usually more effective in individuals who are either overweight or obese.

Helps in gaining a bit of muscle mass

HIIT is perfect for people looking to lose excess weight but, it can also be beneficial if you are looking to gain a bit of muscle mass. Now granted, it is not as effective as going to the gym and lifting weights but, if you are a beginner and not already very active in your daily lifestyle, taking up HIIT has been shown to lead to an increase in muscle in areas such as the legs and trunk. While other areas might show an increase in mass, it is usually the muscles you engage the most when training that will show significant results. Laval University conducted a study that showed HIIT trainees building lean muscle in addition to lowering their body fat percentage. HIIT is so intense that it lowered their bodies' chances of using muscles as fuel and so the end result when their fat had been trimmed away, was a greater definition of lean muscle mass.

The choice is yours

HIIT training offers a versatile workout method that allows trainees to choose their own workouts. Simply pick whatever cardio routine you are comfortable with and voila...you can turn it into an intense, interval workout. From biking to aerobics and jogging, you can choose any exercise that suits your needs.

Good for cardiovascular health

Not many people are cut out for intense training that pushes them beyond their limits and increases their heart and breathing rates to levels they are unfamiliar with. With HIIT, pushing yourself to said levels is made much easier with the introduction of short recovery intervals that come just when you've reached your max out point. This is good for maintain cardiovascular health, from good blood circulation to overall heart health. Research has suggest that HIIT is especially effective at promoting good heart health in obese and overweight people compared to people with normal weight and blood pressure. The Journal of Strength and Conditioning Research also conducted a study that showed that adding moves such as burpees to your high intensity interval training regimen not only improved your body's oxygen consumption but, it improved heart rate as well.

A healthy challenge

From beginners to seasoned trainees, HIIT offers a challenging training method that pushes your body to new, intense heights and keeps you out of your zone of comfort thus ensuring that you are never bored and your muscles and your body avoids hitting a plateau.

Reduction in blood sugar

Research has shown that HIIT training can effectively lower blood sugar when carried out for periods of more than 10 weeks. More than 45 studies have been conducted and they showed that HIIT reduced the level of sugar in the blood while improving the resistance of insulin. This is especially beneficial for people dealing with type 2 diabetes. It is also said to help lower the chances of individuals developing diabetes. Another study conducted on individuals with type-2 diabetes revealed that after four months of high intensity interval training, their VO2 max increased. This means that their bodies could consume more oxygen and thus, burn fat faster while improving their glycemic control.

Effective anti-aging workout

In 2012, at the European Society of Cardiology, a paper was presented citing a direct relationship between life expectancy and physical activity. The paper suggested that exercise activates an anti-aging enzyme called Telomerase and so high intensity interval training would likely increase the levels of said hormone significantly thus, slowing down the effects of aging. According to the paper, HIIT also reduces the expression of p53, a protein that triggers premature aging. Some added anti-aging benefits would also include improved libido and reduction of the appearance of wrinkles and fine lines.

HIIT also balances out very important hormones

Ghrelin is a hormone that causes long-term weight gain as well as eating habits that are more short-term. It is often the "hunger hormone". Made is the stomach, ghrelin is said to be the only hormone that is capable of stimulating the appetite and so, it is the main culprit for unhealthy cravings be it sugar, salt or fried. Ghrelin can also slow down the usage of fat in your body and is released as part of the response to stressful moments which is why many people tend to overeat when they are under a lot of emotional stress. Associate Professor Jeffrey Zigman of UT Southwestern Medical Center explained that raised levels of ghrelin in the body served as logical explanations for people who become obese's unusual eating patterns. He explained that many obese or overweight people are also largely exposed to psychological stress hence the sudden food cravings.

The opposite of this hormone is Leptin or, "the starvation hormone" as it gives the feeling of being "full." When the levels of leptin in your body are balanced, your body is able to maintain sufficient levels of energy and not exceed its limit. This keeps cell function and weight management well balanced and efficient. In the beginning as you gain weight, leptin levels rise and you feel full. But, should you ignore the feeling and continue to supply your body with excess food, it become resistant to leptin thus, leading to weight gain. As individuals take up HIIT training, the levels of ghrelin and leptin in the body are balanced out over time thus, curbing their bodies' cravings for unhealthy food while also stimulating response to leptin which will help them figure out when they have reached their limit.

More enjoyable

Exercise physiologist, Tom Holland has suggested that high intensity interval training is more exciting and enjoyable compared to steadier and lower intensity training. Scientific studies have also backed up this claim, suggesting that people prefer more rigorous and lively training methods to continuous, slower paced exercise. This is important, especially for individuals looking for an exercise regimen to stick to in order to shed excess weight.

There many more health benefits that come with a regular HIIT regimen and many people are sold on the effectiveness of this training method. Despite being so popular and having so many benefits, however, HIIT training is not without its challenges. There are some myths surrounding this popular training method and here are a selection of them that have since been debunked.

Chapter 4: How To Get Started

HIIT is only recommended for people who can sustain cardio aerobic exercises. It's advisable for people who can do 20-30 minutes of cardio. If you can't sustain this phase yet, it is advisable to work on your cardio first before trying HIIT. Forcing your body to perform high intensity training can lead to serious problems such as difficulty in breathing and cramps.

On the other hand, if you do fairly well in cardio exercises, and you decide it's time to take your training one notch higher, HIIT is for you. The strategy for beginners is 10:20, meaning 10 seconds of intense workout followed by 20 seconds low intensity workout or rest. The goal is to rest twice as long as your workout period, so that your body won't easily burn out.

Resting allows the body to adapt to the new routine and recover.

Here are samples of beginner workouts that you can start on:

TIME	ACTIVITY
4 Minutes	Warm-up:
	Jog (2-3 rounds)
	Bend over toe touch
	Leg swings (Front & Back)
	Hip Rotation
30 seconds	Jumping Jacks
1 minute	Rest
40 seconds	Bend-over
1 minute	Rest
30 seconds	Sit/Ups
1 minute	Rest
	**Repeat Warm-Up set for 4minutes to cool down the body

HIIT Level 1 *Repeat each set (30:1) 4 times.

TIME	ACTIVITY
5minutes	WARM-UP
	Jog
	Jump Jacks
	Stretching
60 seconds	Sprint
2minutes	Walk
30 seconds	Sprint
2minutes	Walk
60 seconds	Sprint
2 minutes	Walk
	**Repeat Warm-Up routine for 5minutes

TIME	ACTIVITY
5 minutes	WARM UP
	Jog
	Jump Rope
	Stretching
60 seconds	Fast Cycling
90 seconds	Slow Cycling
60 seconds	Fast Cycling
90 seconds	Slow Cycling
60 seconds	Fast Cycling
90 seconds	Slow Cycling
**Repeat Warm Up	for 5minutes**

HIIT Level 2 * Repeat each set 3 times

HIIT Level 3 *Repeat for 4 cycles each

In order for beginners to sustain HIIT training, the intensity level of the workout should be gradually increased. They should start on a program they are comfortable doing, then increase to mid-level HIIT requiring them to exert more effort. The last stage is an all-out program, pushing the person to his/her limit.

Chapter 5: The Tabata Method

One of the ways in which you can perform HIIT is through the Tabata method. The Tabata offers you the same benefits as any other cardio workout. However, the efficiency of the method is higher than normal cardiovascular exercises and workouts. For starters, the Tabata method can be exercised in a few minutes to get results, as opposed to normal exercises which require hours of exercise daily.

How Did it Start?

The Tabata method was founded by a Japanese scientist. Izumi Tabata worked in the department of physiology in Japan with his fellow colleagues. They decided to study intensity training by drawing a comparison between high intensity training and moderate intensity training.

Tabata conducted tests on two separate groups of athletes, with one group exercising at moderate intensity and another group exercising at high intensity. Both workouts were designed to be interval training workouts.

Group 1 consisted of athletes training with workouts of moderate intensity. The intensity was measured to be 70%. They exercised five days a week for six weeks, and each session lasted an hour.

Group 2 consisted of athletes training with workouts of high intensity. They worked out for four days per week, for a total period of six weeks. Each session lasted 4 minutes. Each session consisted of intervals of intense training at 170% for 20 seconds and rest for 10 seconds.

Results of the Tabata Experiment

Tabata and his colleagues found a marked difference in the results between the two groups of athletes. Group 1 showed significant increase in their cardiovascular or aerobic systems. At the same time, their anaerobic systems, which consist of muscles, barely showed any improvement.

Group 2, on the other hand, revealed improvement in both the systems of all the athletes in the group. Their aerobic systems showed a significant increase, even in comparison to Group 1. In addition, their anaerobic systems showed a 28% increase.

Conclusion of the Experiment

Thus, the Tabata method seems to have very tangible results as compared to moderate intensity interval workout. Not only does it improve both the systems, it also improves them more than a normal workout routine.

However, like everything under the sun, the Tabata method also has its pros and cons. Before applying the Tabata method to your workout routine, you should be aware of all that it can offer, as well as everything that might go wrong if the proper precautions are not taken.

The Pros and Cons of the Tabata Method

Here, we shall outline all the pros and cons of the Tabata method to see if it is for you. It is advisable to be well-educated on everything about the Tabata method before jumping headlong into it. The promise of tangible results within a short period of time is sure to appeal to the desire within all of us. However, without proper precautions, it might cause more harm than you can foresee.

The Advantages of the Tabata Method

Izumi Tabata's findings have revealed that Tabata training will improve your aerobic system significantly. Moderate intensity interval training improves the aerobic system as well. However, high intensity interval training through the Tabata method improves it much more than normal, moderate intensity training.

At the same time, unlike moderate intensity training, the Tabata method of high intensity interval training also improves the anaerobic system of the individual.

Perhaps, most importantly, the Tabata method of training takes less time than a normal method of training. As seen in the experiment, Group 2 only worked out for 4 days a week, and for only 4 minutes, as opposed to Group 1 who worked out for 5 days a week for one hour each. Thus, the Tabata method of training offers you better results within much less time. Therefore, it is more effective than a normal training routine.

Besides these advantages, Tabata training also increases your rate of metabolism. This results in an after effect which allows you to burn calories even after you finish your training session. A high metabolic rate really helps you to burn calories and fat. Thus, with the Tabata method, you can lose weight faster and get into shape.

Aside from the physical benefits of Tabata training, it also has a psychological benefit. Given the high intensity of the method, Tabata training can actually increase your will power or mental toughness. The intensity required is so draining that it makes the routine quite difficult. The athlete will be very tempted to quit in the beginning. Though the high intensity intervals are only for 20 seconds, they seem very long and can be very torturous for the athlete. If the individual can sustain his enthusiasm for long enough and get through the difficulty the method poses in the beginning, his mental state will also gain strength. His resolve will increase, as will his will power.

The Disadvantages of the Tabata Method

The Tabata method definitely has more benefits than disadvantages. However, it is important to list the cons, as they can potentially affect the athlete's health.

For starters, the high intensity of the Tabata method can be potentially harmful to individuals who are prone to heart attacks or strokes. If you are aware of a family history or a personal history of heart attacks or strokes, or even high blood pressure, it is advisable to get a physical and consult with your doctor to see if your body is capable of withstanding the intensity of the Tabata method. Only step into the intense world of Tabata training if you are absolutely sure of your ability to perform the workout.

Secondly, the Tabata method can also be performed with weights. However, if you are not careful with the method and stance, you can harm yourself significantly with the heavy weights and heavy strain on your muscles. At the same time, any kind of accident, such as the bar slipping from your hands can be very dangerous, given the heavy weights employed in Tabata training. In addition, the athlete should be careful to include adequate warm up as well as cool down sessions while training the Tabata way. Without warm up and cool down, the muscles of the body can suffer damage, as the intensity of the Tabata exercises is very high and requires maximum strain on the muscles. You could suffer muscle tears and sprains if you do not acclimatize your body to the intensity at the beginning of the training session. Ideally, the warm up and cool down sessions should each last between 5 to 10 minutes. This might increase the session duration, but it is well worth the time spent.

Thus, the Tabata method offers many more advantages than disadvantages to the athlete. Not only does it improve the aerobic as well as the anaerobic systems of the body, it also aids in weight loss. In addition, this method of training offers psychological benefits as well. However, the disadvantages of the Tabata method can be quite harmful to the individual physically. If the athlete does not take care to ensure that he exercises carefully, the intensity of this form of HIIT training can severely damage his body. In addition, do not be fooled by the fact that the Tabata method burns fat while you sleep, after the workout. There is a reason why it is a HIIT exercise. The intensity is very high and requires strong will power and dedication to sustain. One cannot expect results without putting in equal efforts. By working "short and hard", the reduced time element is compensated in the phenomenal intensity that the Tabata method demands.

Thus, while the Tabata method does offer very attractive benefits to the athlete, one must be in adequate physical shape to employ the intense training it requires. If not, the normal methods of workout are also enough to keep the individual fit, though it will definitely take longer.

Ultimately, the Tabata method is a very effective way to lose weight and get in shape within a short amount of time, as long as the athlete can sustain high intensity interval training on a regular basis.

How to Plan a Tabata Method Workout

Planning a Tabata method workout requires you to keep certain things in mind. First, the exercise should enable you to workout in intervals. Second, you should be capable of performing the exercises even when you are extremely fatigued.

It is best to concentrate on multi-joint exercises, as they really stress the cardio-respiratory system. In addition, they exercise several muscle groups at the same time, giving you the best results.

To plan out your Tabata workout and keep pace with it, you need a clock that has a second hand. If you really wish to get into the Tabata method, you can also consider investing in an interval timer, which will allow you to workout without worrying about the time.

Ideal Exercises for the Tabata Method

Certain exercises are really suited for the Tabata method. These include the following:

- **Skipping –** If you love skipping, you can incorporate skipping in your exercise routine as well. You can change up the usual skipping routine to make it more intensive by performing knee-up sprints and by doing double unders. In double unders, you allow the rope to pass twice under you per jump. However, skipping can strain your lower limbs. Make sure you wear shoes that absorb shock effectively and ensure that the terrain is not very hard.

- **Sprinting –** This is the easiest exercise and one that most people can do.

Sprinting is also a very versatile exercise and can easily be incorporated into a HIIT routine. Sprinting can be performed anywhere, be it the beach, a road or even a garden. Sprint intensely for 20 seconds and then walk at a relaxed pace for 10 seconds. Repeat this routine 8 to 10 times and you have the perfect Tabata method HIIT workout.

- **Rowing Ergometer** – If you have a programmable timer attached to a rowing machine, it makes a very sound Tabata method exercise. Strive to maintain the distance that you cover in each set, or even try to beat your average distance each time. However, ensure that your rowing technique is proper to prevent any injuries due to the intensity of the workout.

These are only three ideal exercises that fit into the Tabata method routine. You can improvise other exercises to fit into the framework of a Tabata method HIIT routine.

A typical Tabata method routine lasts at least 4 minutes. These four minutes are comprised of 20 seconds of intense training and 10 seconds of rest repeated 8 to 10 times. Thus, as long as you can incorporate intervals of intense training and rest, you can convert any exercise into a Tabata method routine.

Tabata Method Workouts

Basic Workout on a Treadmill

Most people prefer to use the treadmill to get their daily exercise. The Tabata method can also be applied to a treadmill by varying the speed at which you run or walk. A basic treadmill workout would look as follows:

- Warm up for 1 minute by walking steadily, and then jogging lightly on the treadmill

- Increase the speed to your maximum possible intensity and run as hard as you can for 20 seconds

- Return to jogging at a slower speed for 10 seconds

- Resume intense running for another 20 seconds

- Jog again for 10 seconds to allow recovery

- Run as hard as you can for another 20 seconds

- Jog lightly for 10 seconds

- Do the final sprint for 20 seconds

- Return to jogging lightly for 10 seconds

- Cool down by slowing bringing down your speed to a comfortable walk

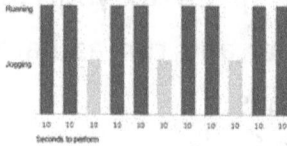

This exercise can be performed by anybody with access to a treadmill. In the absence of a treadmill, you can also sprint on the road while maintaining the timing and the full intensity of the exercise. However, this exercise does not sufficiently exercise all the remaining muscle groups of your body.

For even more effective Tabata method exercises, read the below given workouts as well.

In a Crunch?

For exercisers in a crunch, here's a Tabata method routine that guarantees the same results with limited resources. You can perform these in a deserted office room, hotel room or in someone else's home. They require no equipment other than an interval timer or a clock with a second hand.

The routine goes this way:

- Warm Up

- Pull Ups – 8 rounds with 10 second rest intervals

- Push Ups – 8 rounds with 10 second rest intervals

- Sit Ups – 8 rounds with 10 second rest intervals

- Squats – 8 rounds with 10 second rest intervals

- Cool Down

You do not need anything other than your body to perform this workout. It is perfect for people who are always on the move and do not always have access to a well-equipped gym. Even those who do enjoy the comforts of a gym, can incorporate this routine twice or thrice a week, as it is really effective despite its apparent simplicity.

Crossfit Training

In this cross fitness Tabata workout routine, we mesh five different kinds of exercises to ensure that various muscle groups in your body get exercised. The exercise goes as follows:

- Warm up routine

- Rowing for 20 seconds with a 10 second rest interval for 8 sets

- 1 minute rest interval

- Squats for 20 seconds with a 10 second rest interval for 8 sets

- 1 minute rest interval

- Pull Ups for 20 seconds with a 10 second rest interval for 8 sets

- 1 minute rest interval

- Push Ups for 20 seconds with a 10 second rest interval for 8 sets

- 1 minute rest interval

- Sit Ups for 20 seconds with a 10 second rest interval for 8 sets

- Cool down routine

The entire duration of the workout should come to about 24 minutes, with 4 minutes per exercise intercepted by a 1 minute rest interval between various exercises.

This exercise will provide excellent results, as various muscle groups are exercised simultaneously. In addition, if you keep exercising one particular muscle or muscle group, it gets habituated to the exercise and becomes immune to it. By varying the muscles being used, you ensure that no muscle group has the chance to become habituated to a certain kind of exercise, thus promoting results.

Thus, the Tabata method can be applied to a multitude of exercises by transforming them into interval training workouts. No matter where you are, and whether or not you have access to gym equipment, you can exercise with the Tabata method daily using these different workout routines.

Summary Tabata Workout

Chapter 6: High-Intensity Interval Training

Exercise alone is not effective for long-term weight management, mainly because when we exercise, we eat more. In other words, our brain senses a mismatch between energy expenditure and intake, and our appetite increases to compensate for this mismatch.[23]

Also, most people tend to reduce daytime activity when exercising regularly. Studies have shown that if we exercise in the mornings for, say, an hour, we tend to be less active for the rest of the day. Most of us who exercise regularly are not aware of this subtle tendency to move less on the days we exercise. We do, however, notice the increase in appetite that often occurs after moderate aerobic exercise.

Exercise also increases the stress hormone cortisol. If our goal is to increase lean body mass and reduce fat, excessive exercise may be counterproductive because it elevates cortisol levels. Chronically elevated cortisol levels lead to increased fat storage and muscle breakdown—the opposite of what we want.[24]

Another factor to consider is that exercise causes repetitive use injuries. It goes without saying that if we get injured we can't exercise, but most of us prefer to stick to the same regimen day in and day out. Whether it's weightlifting or running, the risk of repetitive use injury increases with time spent exercising. Each year as many as 70% of runners, for example, will take time off from training due to injury.

To avoid the ravages of cortisol and reduce the risk of injuries, I recommend leisurely walks of about 30 to 60 minutes each day.

During the maintenance phase of an intermittent fast, I recommend high-intensity interval training two to three times each week along with the daily, leisurely walks.

Strategically-Timed Exercise

Strategically timed exercise is nothing more than timing exercise to optimize the hormonal effects of intermittent fasting. For beginners, I recommend easy walks at the beginning of the fasting period. There are two reasons for this. The first is that outdoor walks reduce the stress hormone cortisol.[25] Easy walks, preferably done in a natural setting, limit the cortisol elevations caused by fasting. The second reason I recommend walks is that the compensatory increases in appetite are not as large with walking as compared to other forms of vigorous physical activity.[26] I should emphasize that these are leisurely walks, not power walks, hikes, or light jogs. These walks are done at a conversational pace, a speed at which you could talk without pausing to catch your breath. Leisurely walks lasting thirty to sixty minutes, five to six days each week, minimize cortisol spikes observed with other strenuous physical activities.

You can walk at any time, but I find that most people prefer to walk at the beginning of their fasting period.

After the first two weeks of fasting and leisurely walks, I recommend beginning high-intensity interval training. The best time to perform high-intensity interval training is at the end of the fast.

How to Get Started with High-Intensity Training

After you've completed the two-week induction fast, you're ready to begin the next phase with high-intensity interval training.

To start, select a mode of exercise that you enjoy. Most people find running to be the most convenient choice because it requires no additional equipment other than a good pair of running shoes. Indoor stationary cycles are another good option and are easier on the knees. In fact, many of the studies on the benefits of high-intensity interval training use stationary cycles that measure power output during the high-intensity phase of the exercise intervals. My favorite choice for performing high-intensity interval training is an indoor rowing machine such as the C2 Concept Rower. Indoor rowers, or "ergometers" as they are sometimes called, provide a total body workout by working the upper body, core, and lower body during the pulling and recovery phases of the row. Many feature a display that gives you detailed information about your heart rate and power output.

Another factor to consider is that, whichever mode you choose, you must exercise at an intensity of at least 80% of your maximum heart rate. Most people find that running or sprinting is the easiest way to achieve that intensity. If you are new to indoor cycling or rowing, you may find it difficult to attain that level of intensity until you have mastered the use of your machine.

The bottom line is that you should select a mode of exercise that you enjoy. Even the most efficient exercise machine won't help if you don't enjoy using it.

How To Calculate Your Training Heart Rate

The formula that is often used in research studies to calculate working heart rate is the Karvonen formula[27].

Target Heart Rate = ((max HR – resting HR) × %Intensity) + resting HR

Maximum heart rate (max HR) can be estimated by subtracting your age from 220.

Resting heart rate (resting HR) is calculated by measuring your heart rate at rest. The best time to measure your resting heart rate is within 30 minutes of waking.

Percent Intensity refers to your target exercise intensity. For high-intensity interval training the recommended intensity is 80%-90% of your maximum heart rate.

Let's consider an example of how to use this formula. Let's say that a thirty-year-old male plans to begin high-intensity interval training at an intensity of 80%. His estimated maximum heart rate would be

190 (220-30). Let's further suppose that his resting pulse rate taken within thirty minutes of waking is 70. Using the Karvonen formula, we would have the following equation:

$$((190 - 70)) \times .80 + 70 = 166$$

To benefit from high-intensity interval training in this example, the target heart rate during the high-intensity interval would be 166 beats per minute.

Don't expect to get your heart rate to the required intensity within the first few intervals. For most, it takes about five minutes of intense exercise to reach the target rate.

How To Structure Your High-Intensity Interval Training Sessions

Once you've selected your exercise mode and calculated your training heart rate, you're ready to begin your first high-intensity interval training session.

There are two helpful tools you might want to use.

The first is a heart rate monitor. There are many models to choose from, and prices range anywhere from $30.00 at the low end to as much as $400.00 at the high end. My favorite is the Wahoo Fitness monitor, which is compatible with most smartphones.

The second tool is an interval timer. Here again there are many choices. There are dozens of smartphone apps to choose from. My favorite is Seconds Pro. There are also stand-alone interval timers such as the GymBoss interval timer (www.gymboss.com) that allow you to program work time, recovery time, and the total number of intervals.

Next, decide how you'd like to structure your interval sessions. The protocol that works best for beginners is the 8:12 protocol: exercise hard for eight seconds, and then rest for twelve seconds.[28] Repeat this cycle for twenty minutes. When done this way, you'll complete a total of sixty rounds of 8:12 in twenty minutes. Add to this a five-minute warm-up and cool-down period, and your total time spent exercising amounts to thirty minutes.

To summarize, you'll do your 8:12 interval sessions for twenty minutes three times each week and your leisurely walks at least five times each week.

Chapter 7: Hiit With Cycling

To those who find running not as fun, cycling might come as a more interesting option. Not only will your cardio be developed from this routine, your quads and hips will become stronger too. Since the core will also be engaged, it is highly likely that sagging bellies will get smaller, and the abs will get toned.

Unlike running, however, cycling is less complicated when it comes to interval training. The only variants will come from revolutions per minute (RPM), seconds, and heart rate. Be sure to have a heart rate monitor ready before exercising to have an efficient way of measuring your performance.

You can do this with a stationary bike or with a regular one, but the former is more ideal because controlled resistance is essential. This will add intensity to your workout, hence faster results. If, however, you don't have or access to any, then you may have to mix your workout with bodyweight exercises in between cycling intervals.

Training Guide

Again, the following routines will be categorized by level to help your body gradually adapt to higher intensity workouts. Beginners are encouraged to start with the first level. However, if you find it too easy, you are free to skip to higher levels.

Level 1 : Basic Interval Cycling

There's not much to take note from this interval exercise because it will mainly focus on how much you can do without resistance, making it highly ideal for those new to cycling.

Like everything else, start your routine with a warm-up. Cycle at a comfortable pace for three minutes, and keep your heart rate at a 65% maximum.

Once your muscles are warm and ready, explode and cycle as fast as you can for twenty seconds. Then for ten seconds, slow down to a comfortable pace and recover. Repeat this for eight rounds, then cool down for three minutes.

You can add intensity by extending the fast-cycling interval to thirty seconds or more. However, if your body still needs to adapt to this workout, you can lengthen your recovery period to twenty or thirty seconds.

Do this for one week before transitioning to level two.

Level 2 : 120 and Up

This is where you will have to focus on your RPM, and this is where the intensity will come from.

Again, start with a warm-up. Target and maintain the same heart rate as in level one. Then for thirty seconds, pedal as hard as you can, and work on keeping your RPM at 120 or higher. Rest for thirty seconds by slowing down, then repeat until you finish eight rounds. Once you're done, cool down for three minutes before hopping off your bike.

The intensity of this workout will rely on the 120 RPM, so you will have to focus on **not** going down that number. If this is a bit too easy for you, then target a higher RPM.

Keep to this routine for two weeks.

Level 3 : 1 KM Cycle

This is where distance and speed meets, so your body needs to be highly adapted to cycling before opting for this level. If you think one week for level two is not enough, feel free to add another week for the workout.

Start this routine with a three-minute warm-up. For the high intensity interval, cover 1 KM by cycling as fast as you can. Just like in level two, your ideal RPM is 120. If you can manage a higher number, then do so, but what's important is to not go down this benchmark. Recover by cycling at a comfortable pace, until your heart rate reaches a 75% maximum. Complete five rounds of this, then cool down for three minutes.

Do this routine for two weeks.

Level 4 : 110 Pyramid Cycle

Resistance will come to play in this level, so if you managed to accomplish the first three with a regular bike, you may need to find or invest on a stationary one to accommodate your final hurdle.

As usual, start the routine with a warm-up. Don't forget to reach a 65% maximum heart rate before jumping in the main exercise.

Start the main exercise by reaching and maintaining 110 RPM for thirty seconds. Increase the resistance by a notch without compromising your pace, and keep it for thirty seconds. Up the resistance once more, and repeat this process until you cannot maintain the 110 RPM anymore. Take a three-minute rest after.

Start again from the top until you complete three rounds. Maintain this workout for two weeks.

Training Schedule

The cycling HIIT program will take more weeks than running. You have more muscles at work here, and you'll need to adapt each to the exercise. Again, this is a schedule suited for fitness newbies. Feel free to adjust it according to your capabilities if level one is too easy for you.

	Mon	Tue	Wed	Thu	Fri	Sat	Sun
Week 1	Level 1	Rest	Level 1	Rest	Level 1	Rest	Stretch
Week 2	Level 2	Rest	Level 2	Rest	Level 2	Rest	Stretch
Week 3	Level 2	Rest	Level 2	Rest	Level 2	Rest	Stretch

	With 135 RPM		With 135 RPM		With 135 RPM		
Week 4	Level 3	Rest	Level 3	Rest	Level 3	Rest	Stretch
Week 5	Level 3 With 140 RPM	Rest	Level 3 With 140 RPM	Rest	Level 3 With 140 RPM	Rest	Stretch
Week 6	Level 4	Rest	Level 4	Rest	Level 4	Rest	Stretch
We	Lev	Re	Lev	Re	Lev	Re	Stret

ek 7	el 4	st	el 4	st	el 4	st	ch
	With 115 RPM		With 115 RPM		With 115 RPM		

Reminders

Basically, the reminders in the previous chapter applies to the cycling HIIT program. Where the two differs is in the type of stretches that should be done every Sunday. The muscle groups that will be most worked out in cycling are the quads and the hip flexors. Focus your stretch on those areas, or opt for yoga classes to further relax your lower body.

Chapter 8: Fat Burning Myths Exposed

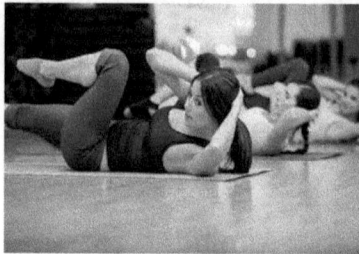

Each new generation of individuals who want to lose weight falls prey to the fat burning myths that have been around for years and years. Check out these myths:

* Lots of direct stomach work will melt belly fat. All that 800 crunches a day will do is make you good at doing 800 crunches a day. Abdominal muscles are small and weak; they require small amounts of energy to function, even when performing crunches and sit-ups. Just because there's fat surrounding these muscles, doesn't mean forcing these muscles to fold, bend and twist will melt the fat.

* In order to shrink the belly, you must bend, fold and twist. Marketers of gadgets that do this have the masses brainwashed. Did you know that the abs can be tremendously worked without folding, crunching, bending or twisting? Does a competitive sprinter fold, crunch, bend or swivel? Yet wow, look at the abs of any competitive sprinter! Their specialty movement involves a very linear, upright position, yet dang, they have killer abs!

* In order to lose large amounts of fat all over, you must keep the heart rate continually elevated during exercise. Wrong. As you will see later on in this tutorial, exercise that's based on steady pacing is inferior to peak-and-valley style exercise, in which the heart rate soars, then returns close to baseline, repeatedly throughout the session.

* Some people are meant to be large. If this were true, the percentage of obese men and women in developed countries would be nearly the same as it was several generations ago.

* If a person has big bones, their ability to lose weight is limited. Bone diameter has nothing to do with the amount of fat in fat cells. The diameter of bones in an obese person is the same as in a medium weight person of the same height and gender. Though the density of bones varies and is influenced by lifestyle habits, the diameter remains pretty much constant. A "small boned" person can be obese, and a "large boned" person can be very lean.

* The best way to burn fat is with long, long cardio sessions. Marathon athletes are thin, sometimes scary skinny. But they also run 10 to 15 miles a day at a painful pace. During prime time, look at the people on the cardio equipment at your gym, spending lengthy amounts of time pedalling, stepping, plodding along on the treadmill, taking two dance classes in a row. How many are tight and lean?

* **In order to become trim, you must exercise two or three hours a day.** Though competitive athletes train up to six hours a day, they train to outperform everyone else. Optimal fat loss isn't about outperforming everyone else, and does not require more than an hour a day of the right kind of exercise.

* The inner and outer thigh machines will shrink the thighs. **Nope. Not in a million years. Trust me on this.**

* Multiple pregnancies permanently add fat. You won't find this statement in any medical journal.

* Most cases of obesity are caused by medical conditions. Some medications and conditions (e.g., menopause, polycystic ovary syndrome, and hypothyroidism) cause weight gain, but not 100 pounds. Most of the weight gain caused by these conditions is less than 50 pounds, sometimes only 10 or 20. There is a genetic condition (Prader-Willi syndrome) that can cause extreme obesity, but it's estimated that only one in 5,000 morbidly obese individuals has it.

* Fat-burning comes in a pill. If this were true, few people would be hefty. "Fat burner" pills, at the most, elevate metabolism to such a small degree that it's negligible.

* Crash dieting is a good solution to obesity. Diets with non-sustainable rules and prohibitions may work in the short term, but science has proven, time and time again, that severe caloric restriction and other gimmicky features such as cutting out food groups will ultimately lead to failure and gaining the lost weight back.

* The secret to weight loss is counting calories. This may work for people whose brains are hardwired for meticulous tracking of everything that occurs in their lives (they are often accountants, financial planners, engineers, computer programmers, etc.). But most people will tire of this approach or become discouraged.

Chapter 9: Pros And Cons

Efficiency

Perhaps the top reason for the appeal of HIIT is efficiency. The trade-off between time and progress is better than a lot of other exercise routines. Less time spent with more progress means it can be a sufficient exercise for people who just want to be fit despite their busy schedules.

Several studies have concluded that shorter interval training sessions let the individual achieve more compared to longer steady-pace sessions. For example, 15 minutes of HIIT done thrice a week garners more progress than 1 hour of steady pace jogging on a treadmill. This kind of efficiency doesn't stop at fat and calorie burning. In a study done in 2011 by the American College of Sports Medicine, it was found that 2 weeks of HIIT improves a person's aerobic capacity the same level as 6 to 8 weeks of endurance training.

Burns More Fat

HIIT doesn't only burn more calories. It also burns more fat. Moreover, HIIT will activate your body's repair mode and turn it into overdrive. This is because of the intense exertion you're doing. What does this mean for fat and calorie burning? Well, that means you will not only be burning calories during the workout but an increased metabolism means you will also continue to burn them throughout the 24 hours after.

Weight Loss, Not Muscle

When you go into a weight-reducing diet, you'll find that it's difficult to not reduce your muscle mass as you strip off fat. Steady pace cardio workout has been shown to encourage muscle loss. On the other hand, HIIT has been shown to help preserve muscle mass and ensure that majority of the weight lost is from fat. HIIT is a good workout to pair with diet.

No Equipment Needed

You can perform HIIT without equipment. While there are people who do HIIT with treadmills, exercise bikes, jumping ropes and rowboats, no-equipment exercises can work just as well as long as they get your heart rate up as fast. Some examples are sprints, fast jogs, fast feet, high knees or plyometric exercises like jumping lunges or burpees.

There are even times when equipment may hinder the effectiveness of HIIT. For example, dumbbells may slow down your heart rate gain. The muscle you want to push is your heart, not your biceps.

Can be Done Anywhere

Going to the gym for HIIT is also optional. You can do it anywhere since you don't need any equipment and it is not time-intensive. The concept of HIIT is really simple and once your specific program is laid out, it will be easy to follow. You will have no problem adapting to whatever constraints you have on both time and space.

Challenging

As mentioned before, HIIT is not easy. You will be pushing yourself to the max in the high intensity periods because of how short the durations are. So this is something you can't do while watching TV, reading a book or chitchatting with a friend. Those who love to seek new challenges, especially fitness buffs would love HIIT. It will push you to your limits, but the pace won't let you get bored.

Cons

While the above characteristics really make HIIT appealing, it is important to mention that it's not perfect. There are still cons to HIIT, such as the following:

You work more in shorter time, but that means higher intensity and volume of training. Risk of injury is higher in these states of exercise.

As mentioned before, it is not recommended for everyone. You can't just jump in right into HIIT as your body might not be able to handle maximum exertion.

HIIT is not sufficient in training for specified events, such as a triathlon. You'd still need the specific training for endurance events.

Next...

Now, you have been acquainted with the advantages and disadvantages of HIIT. In the next chapter, you will learn about the different benefits studies have found one can get from HIIT.

Chapter 10: Top Hiit Exercises

There are literally hundreds of exercises out there that you can apply to HIIT training and be used to burn some serious fat. You can keep it simple by using just a treadmill, a skipping rope, a bicycle or any cardio machine you may find at a gym, or you can put together mixed routines that change at each interval and throw in some dumbbells or a kettle bell and work muscles too.

To make sure that you get the full benefits of HIIT training you want to use your whole body throughout a workout to up that heart rate and get the after burn effect. For that reason we won't be discussing bicep curls or kickbacks. Instead, we will focus on compound exercises that get you closer to your VO2 max. In this chapter, we'll provide the technique for the best HIIT movements to burn fat and get super lean. Take the time to learn proper technique in order to avoid injuries while working out.

Upper body

Rows

Start standing with your dumbbells in your hands at your sides. Bend forward from the hips but keep your back straight! Allow the weight to hang down toward the ground in front of you. Pull your elbows back close to your waist from this position. At the top of the movement squeeze your back muscles together and then lower the weights again. Make sure your back is nearly parallel to the floor during this exercise. You want to work back muscles not your shoulders. You can use dumbbells or a single kettlebell or even a bar for this one. This will work your back and arms.

Pushups

Start lying face down on the floor with your hands next to your shoulders and your toes on the floor. Keeping your back and legs totally straight push your body off the floor until your arms are straight. Lower your body slowly to the floor by bending your elbows while keeping back and legs straight. Keep your elbows fairly close to your waist as you do this. If it is too hard then you can try keeping your knees on the floor as your body's pivot point instead of your feet. Regardless don't let your hips sag to the floor or stick your butt out to the sky. This will work your chest, shoulders and arms.

Lower Body

Dumbbell Squats

Stand with dumbbells at your sides in your hands. Place your feet at about the same distance apart as your hips and turn your toes slightly out. Slowly bend your knees while you push out your backside. Go as low as you can comfortably or to where your thighs become parallel to the ground. Push back up to starting position. Push through your heels not your toes; your heels should hold more of your weight. Don't let your back hunch forward at any point. Keep your backside stuck out as far as you can behind you. This can be done with a single kettlebell in front, a barbell in front resting across the upper arms or behind the neck resting across the shoulders.

Lunges

Start standing with dumbbells in your hands at your sides and your feet shoulder width. Step forward with one foot and bend that knee as you lower your body. Your other knee should almost touch the ground. Push with your front foot to stand up again and bring your back foot forward next to your other foot the same as your starting position. Repeat but swap sides. If this is too hard don't use any weights or you can increase them if you want to. Keep your back straight.

Core/Abs

Sit Ups

Start lying on your back, with your knees bent and your feet flat on the ground. Place your hands by your sides. Pull in your belly button so that your entire back gets to touch the ground and roll up until you are sitting upright. Reverse back down. You can put your feet under a couch or something that will achieve the same to stabilize yourself while you perform the sit up if it is too hard to do normally. You can also take one leg off the ground and put it up in the air if you want an extra challenge.

Leg Lifts

Lay on your back the same as with the sit ups. Keep your hands beside you, your feet together and your legs straight. Now, while keeping your legs straight, lift both of them so that they are at a right angle to the floor. Keep your back touching the floor. Lower your legs slowly back to the floor. If you have any strain in your lower back you can try putting your hands under your backside. If this is too hard you can lower one leg at a time or bend your knees so that your lower leg is parallel with the floor when raised. If it becomes too easy try lifting your upper back off the floor at the same time.

Compound Exercises

Burpees

Start in a standing position. No weights. Squat down and put your hands on the ground. Next jump your feet backward so that you're in the push up position. Jump them forward again into the squat position and then jump once on the spot and you are back at the start position. If this exercise is too hard you can try stepping back and forward instead of jumping. For an additional challenge try jumping onto a box or step and back down, rather than jumping on the spot. You can increase the height of the box or step.

Kettlebell / Dumbbell Swing

Start in a standing position with your feet out wide and toes slightly outward. You should be holding a kettle bell or dumbbell in front of you in both hands. Next bend your knees and push out your backside. Keep your back straight and your abs tight and swing the kettle back like you are trying to grab the wall behind you. Now stand, push your pelvis forward and swing the kettle with your arms straight until they are holding the kettle straight out in front of you at head height. You are not lifting with your arms. You should be using your hips and legs for the hard work. You will be doing this quite explosively and using momentum. Increase or decrease weights to vary the challenge.

Dumbbell Clean and Press

Start standing, feet shoulder width apart and two dumbbells on the ground in front of you. Keeping your back straight, bend your knees and hip joints and pick up the dumbbells with your arms straight. Start straightening your legs and pulling the weight from the ground. Move your pelvis forward and raise your shoulders and shrug them, using the momentum to pull the weight up as high as you can but keep it close to your body. Rotate your palms so they face up and your elbows so they point forward and bring your body under the weights so they sit at your shoulder level. Stand up and push the dumbbells over your head. Lower them back to the floor without hunching your back and keeping your pelvis back. Increase or decrease weight to vary the challenge. You can use a barbell for this exercise too.

Chapter 11: High Intensity Interval Training For Beginners

High intensity interval training might be hard for you if you are not an enthusiastic exerciser. Even doing HIIT drills for beginners might be a challenge for you. But as the session started, you would have a better endurance and the eagerness to take your workout routine to the next level.

The following exercises will help you burn your fat and tone your muscle. Even without the thrilling effect of extreme, full out effort phases, you will get the benefits of HIIT and make you feel ready for a more intense training.

Yet, an HIIT routine for beginners doesn't have very effective exercises. That is why you should do this routine 5 to 6 days a week.

Warm Up Exercises

These Cardio warm up exercises should be done for at least 4 minutes. It would warm your muscles and make them ready to work.

Crossover Toe Touch Stretch

Stand up straight. Then, cross your right leg in front and over your left leg. Bend over to touch your feet for five seconds. Balance yourself while feeling the burn in your leg. Return to upright position and uncross legs. Alternate legs and do the same procedure. Repeat motion for a total of 30 reps with 15 reps on each leg.

Standing Crisscross Crunches

Stand up straight. Bring down your right elbow to meet your left knee at about hip level. Hold this position for a few seconds. Then, repeat the procedure for the other elbow and knee. Alternate your elbows back and forth through the entire phase.

Torso Rotations

Have an inflatable ball. Sit on a mat. Lean back slightly. Bend your knees. Hold the ball with two hands. Rotate the ball with your arms stretched.

High Kicks

Raise your knee above waist level. Extend your leg. Chamber and then straighten it out. Snap it right back into another chamber. Repeat the process for the desired times.

Leg Swings, Front to Back

Hold on to the wall with one arm. The wall should be at your side, not in your front. Swing your leg backward as high as you can. Keep your hips loose and relax your body the entire period.

HIIT Exercises

This portion of the routine involves the core, upper body, and lower body. You will work for 20 seconds and pause for 10 seconds before you repeat the procedure for two times. Move to the next exercise after that. Have two minutes of rest after doing all five exercises.

But having rest doesn't mean you will lay yourself on the bed or sit back and relax. You need to keep on moving by walking, marching in place, doing jumping jacks or stretching. Repeat the HIIT exercises after having a two-minute active rest.

Jumping Jacks

Stand up straight, your arms at your side. Slightly bend your knees and jump. While in air, spread your legs and raise your arms. Land on forefoot with legs apart and your arms over your head. Jump again while bringing down your arms and returning legs to the midline. Your arms and legs should be in the original position as you land on the forefoot. Repeat the exercise.

Squat/ Crosskick

Stand up straight. Your feet should be shoulder-width apart. Stretch your arms apart. Chin up, lift your chest and tighten your abdominal muscles. Squat until thighs are parallel to the floor. Hold this position for a few seconds, then stand upright with the heels pressed to the floor. Keep the rump muscles tight. Stand up and kick with one leg. If you use the left leg, kick on the right side. If you use the right leg, kick at the opposite side. Land your foot in the same place and squat again. Use the other leg for kicking.

Traveling Push Ups

Do the normal push-up. Then, walk your hands over about 6 inches to the left and do another push-up. Repeat the procedure for a couple of times before you travel back to the right.

Crossover Crunches

Lie on your back. Bend your knees. Cross your right leg over your left leg. Your right ankle should rest on your left knee. Hold the side of your head just behind the ears. Gently twist your torso. Then, reach for your left elbow to your right knee. Exhale as you stand up. Inhale as you go back to the starting position. Repeat the procedure.

Fingertip to Toe Jacks

Lift your leg slowly for you to reach your toes each time. Lift the leg higher quickly until you are actually hopping back and forth from leg to leg with only one foot on the ground at a time. While doing this, raise your one hand while the other hand is going down. Alternate your hands while repeating the process.

Sample Beginner Workouts:

TIME	ACTIVITY
4 Minutes	Warm-up
	Jog (2-3 rounds)
	Bend-over toe touch
	Leg swings (Front & Back)
	Hip Rotation
30 seconds	Jumping Jacks
1 minute	Rest
40 seconds	Bend-over
1 minute	Rest
30 seconds	Sit-Ups
1 minute	Rest
	**Repeat Warm-Up set for 4minutes to cool down the body

HIIT Level 1 *Repeat each set (30:1) 4 times.

TIME	ACTIVITY
5minutes	WARM-UP
	Jog
	Jump Jacks
	Stretching
60 seconds	Sprint
2minutes	Walk
80 seconds	Sprint
2minutes	Walk
60 seconds	Sprint
2 minutes	Walk
	**Repeat Warm-Up routine for 5minutes

HIIT Level 2 * Repeat each set 3 times

TIME	ACTIVITY
5 minutes	WARM UP
	Jog
	Jump Rope
	Stretching
60 seconds	Fast Cycling
90 seconds	Slow Cycling
60 seconds	Fast Cycling
90 seconds	Slow Cycling
60 seconds	Fast Cycling
90 seconds	Slow Cycling
**Repeat Warm Up	for 5minutes**

HIIT Level 3 *Repeat for 4 cycles each

In order for beginners to sustain HIIT training, the intensity level of the workout should be gradually increased. They should start on a program they are comfortable doing, then increase to mid-level HIIT requiring them to exert more effort. The last stage is an all-out program, pushing the person to his/her limit.

Chapter 12: Beginner Level Hiit Workouts

Ok, now that we've covered the basics, we will cover 100 different HIIT exercises that you can mix and match, depending on your HIIT fitness level. In this chapter, we'll kick off your HIIT campaign with beginner level workouts.

Since this book is all about HIIT workouts that you can do just about anywhere at anytime, I won't cover weight lifting exercises. It can be quite impractical and cumbersome to bring your barbells and dumbbells on your out of town or out of the country on vacation. As such, they're disqualified for the purposes of this book.

The exercises included in this book are all bodyweight centered and are classified into 2 groups: pure bodyweight exercises and suspension exercises, i.e., TRX suspension trainers. The reason I included suspension exercises is that suspension trainers can easily fit in just about any bag and can be used anywhere there's a sturdy overhead bar or door, which will allow you to bring and use it anywhere you go – even when you're on vacation!

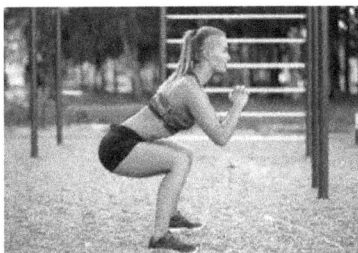

Bodyweight Exercises

Sumo squats: Place your feet slightly wider than hip-width, with your toes pointing outward at an angle of 45 degrees. With your weight resting on your heels, your chest upright, and your back flat, bring yourself down just until your thighs are about parallel to the floor. Use your butt muscles – a.k.a. glutes – as well as your quads (thigh muscles) to bring yourself back up to the starting position. Perform as many repetitions as fast as you can within your preferred high-intensity interval.

Jumping Jacks: Begin with an upright standing position with feet about hip-width apart and arms to the side. While raising your arms overhead in a sideways manner, jump and spread your feet out to the sides. Jump again to bring your feet back to hip-width stance and your arms back down to the sides. Perform as many repetitions as fast as you can within your preferred high-intensity interval.

Boxer's Punches: Begin by standing upright with your left foot in front of the left, and your hips at a diagonal position facing forward. Assume a boxer's position where your upper arms are parallel to the ground and your forearms perpendicular to it – forming a 90-degree angle at the elbows. Throw a jab with your left hand, then a cross punch with your right hand. As you throw the cross punch, let your upper body rotate at the waist as your right arm crosses over to the center-left. At this point, your bodyweight should be resting on the left foot already and your right back-heel lifting off the ground. Return both arms back to your body and shifting your weight back to the right foot and returning the heel to the floor – the starting position. Perform as many repetitions as fast as you can within your preferred high intensity interval and for the next high-intensity interval, reverse the position so that you jab with your right and cross with your left. As you punch, never let your arms lock out straight at the elbow. Stop short of locking out the elbows to minimize risks for elbow overextension injuries.

Kneeling Pushups: Kneel on the floor and put both hands on the ground at about shoulder width. Keeping your lower back and upper body straight, lower your chest to the ground until the point where your elbows form a 90-degree angle. Return to starting position.

Countertop Pushups: Stand about 3 to 4 feet in front of a counter or table top (make sure they're sturdy enough to support your weight). Lean forward and put both hands at shoulder-width apart on the edge of the counter top or table while keeping your whole body straight. Lower your body until your elbows form a 90-degree angle before pushing yourself back up, stopping short of locking your elbows (stopping at this point instead of locking your elbows at the top minimizes the risk for elbow injuries).

Negative Pushups: Assume the normal push up position on the floor, with your arms nearly straight – elbows stopping short of locking out – and your whole body straight. Bring your chest down to the ground very slowly – as in painfully slow – until it touches the ground. Let your knees relax and touch the floor and bring yourself up to the starting position by lifting up your torso – with your knees on the ground as a fulcrum point – before lifting the legs and forming a straight line with your body to perform the next repetition. This is probably the only HIIT exercises where increasing intensity means performing fewer reps as possible because the intensity lies going against gravity.

Butt Kicks: Walk or run in place (running is higher intensity) by kicking the left heel up as far as you can to touch your left butt while keeping your left thigh perpendicular to the floor. Do the same with the right heel.

Triceps Body Dips: With your back to a sturdy chair, bench, or very low table, put both hands on the edge with legs stretched out in front. Bring your butt as low to the floor as you can by bending at the elbows before pushing back up to the starting position.

Lunges To The Side: Rest your body weight on your heels, with your toes facing to the front. Then, make a huge step to the right for a deep side lunge and making sure that your toes never go beyond your toes. Do the same to the left side.

Switching Lunges: Stand up straight and make a forward step with your right leg. Bring your body as low as you can until your right knee's bent at a 90-degree angle and your left (rear) knee is only inches off the floor then push back up to the starting position. On the next rep, do the same with your left foot/leg and remember to keep your upper body straight the whole time. Continue alternating.

Skater Hops: Begin by standing straight with your weight on your left foot and left knee bent. Lift your right leg from off the floor just behind you. Then, bound to your right by pushing off with the left leg and landing on your right foot. This time, it's your left leg that you'll lift off the floor. That's one repetition.

Reverse Switching Lunges: Standing upright and feet at hip-width, keep your hands together on your chest with your elbows bent and extending outside of your shoulders. With your torso staying upright, take a step backward using your right foot and assume a lunging position, and perform a lunge before pushing back to the starting position and repeating with the other foot.

Switching Side X Lunges: With feet hip-width apart and standing upright, put your hands together on your chest and elbows bent and extending out to the shoulders. Take a step back with your left foot but this time, your left foot should cross-over to land behind to the right side of your right foot, and bring your body down with body straight all throughout. Aim to achieve a 90-degree bend at the right knee and let your left knee hover an inch or two above ground. Push to go back to the starting position and do the same with the other leg/foot.

Bodyweight Rows: Grab an overhead bar that can support your body weight with an overhand or pronated grip, and place your feet on an elevated platform like a chair or bench. With your body straight, perform a 45-degree angle with your arms fully extended. Pull your chest towards the bar, keeping your body straight and your feet planted on the platform. Return to starting position and repeat.

Sprints: Just run as fast as you possibly can for the duration of your high-intensity interval.

Carioca: Begin by assuming an athletic stance – your feet about hip-width apart. Run sideways by putting one foot across and in front of the other then behind it. Later on, reverse the directions with the other foot going in front and behind the other.

Stair Flights: Just go up a flight of stairs as fast as you can for the duration of your high-intensity interval. Go down at a relaxed pace as your alternating low intensity interval.

Jump-Assisted Pull-ups: Look for an overhead bar that's about 2 feet at most above your head and that's sturdy enough to support your weight. With your hands on the bar at slightly wider than shoulders, jump while pulling yourself up the bar until your chin is at bar level. Then, lower your body in a gradual and controlled manner.

Running Knee-Ups: Run in place as fast as you can by lifting your knees alternately as high as you can for the duration of your high-intensity interval.

Forward Leaps: Stand upright with feet together. With arms to the side, bring them backwards and bending at the hips (keeping your back straight, leap as far as you can forward, landing on both feet at the middle or forefoot to reduce the impact on your knees.

Box or Bench Jumps: Stand straight with feet at hip-width in front of a sturdy 8-inch-high box or bench that can support your weight. Bend at the knees and hips and jump on the top of the bench or box before jumping back down for the duration of your high-intensity interval.

Mountain Climbers: Assume a regular pushup position with your body straight and core (abs and lower back) engaged and tight. Pull your right knee as close as you can to your chest while keeping your lower back straight, return it to the starting position, and do the same with the left knee, alternating throughout the high- intensity interval.

Side Planks: Lie on your right side and keep your knees straight. Prop your body up using your right forearm and elbow and bring your left hand up until your whole right arm's perpendicular with your upper body. At this point, your body will resemble a letter "T". Contract your abs like you're preparing for a strong punch to the gut and raise our hips so your body will form a straight line from your right ankle up to your shoulders. Maintain the position for the duration of your high-intensity interval before relaxing back to the original position.

TRX SUSPENSION TRAINING

Standing Chest Presses: Standing with feet at shoulder width and back to the TRX's anchor, grab both handles using an overhand grip. Raise both arms in front at shoulder height and lean forward to create a slight diagonal with your body, while keeping your whole body straight from feet to shoulders. Lower your body by bending at the elbows until your chest is along the same lines as your hands before pushing back up to the original position, stopping short of elbow lockout to maintain continuous tension and high intensity.

Suspended Rows: Grab both handles with your hands using a supinated (facing upward) grip and stand straight facing towards the TRX's anchor. With your body straight, lean back at a 45-degree angle or until your arms are nearly straight. Pull your self back to an upright position while keeping your body straight from head to toe. To increase resistance or weight, a step closer to the anchor and lean back further at an angle that's less than 45 degrees.

3D Rows: Perform suspended rows but using 3 different grips all throughout: supinated (palms upward), pronated (palms downward), and palms facing each other.

Inverted Rows: Lie down on the floor directly under the TRX with knees bent and feet planted firmly on the floor. Grasp each of the handles with your palms looking at each other and your arms extended fully. The handles should be at a height where after grasping them and arms fully extended, your body's an inch or two off the floor. Pull your torso up as close as possible to the handles using your elbows and keeping your whole body straight before returning to starting position.

TRX Swings: Stand in front of the TRX's anchor point with feet at a wide-legged stance and grab one handle with each hand using an overhand grip. With your bodyweight resting on your heels, bend at the hips and extend arms in front at about the height of your chest. Rotate your upper body with your left arm extended in front of you and your right arm extended behind. Reverse and do the same on the opposite side.

Suspended Squats: Stand in front of the TRX, facing its anchor point. Hold the handles in front of the waist with both elbows slightly bent at the sides. Perform a squat while holding the TRX's handles in front of you at eye level with arms extended. Return to starting position.

Single Suspension Squat: Slip one foot through the TRX's strap handles – the shin should be parallel to the ground – and stand with the other leg. Perform a squat with only one leg and do the same with the other leg.

Suspended Side-Lunges: Stand in front of the TRX, with feet at shoulder-width and facing its anchor. Hold a handle in each hand at the waist and elbows bended at the side. Plant one foot firmly on the floor and take a huge step to the side by bending at the knee of the other leg. Go back to the starting position and do the same for the other leg.

Gluteus Bridges: Begin by lying on the floor on your back and slip your feet into the handles' cradles. Bring your feet towards your hips to create a 90-degree bend at the knees. Straighten your arms out on your sides and while keeping your upper body straight, lift your hips off the floor until your upper torso has formed a diagonal line. Return to starting position and repeat.

Squat Rows: Begin by holding the handles in front at waist level, with elbows bent at the sides. Extend your arms as you lean back until your hands are at eye level. Perform a squat using the straps of the TRX trainer as support and balance. As you push yourself back up, pull your body using the elbows towards the TRX's anchor point. Try to bring your chest as close to the handles as possible.

Suspended Planks: Assume the regular planking position with your body facing away from the TRX. Slip your feet into the TRX's handle stirrups and your feet facing the floor. Lift your body with your elbows and forearms as you would with regular planks and hold the position for as long as you can without breaking good form, i.e., straight body.

Curly Crunches: Using an underhand grip, grab both handles and lie on the floor with your arms straight up in the air at your front, feet flat, and knees bent. Maintain a very tight core, curl your arms while simultaneously lifting your back and shoulders off the ground. Return to starting position and repeat.

Chapter 13: Working Out Beyond The Bike - Let's Build Some Muscle

In the previous chapter, we showed you how to do HIIT using your bike. That bike routine is perfect for improving your cardio-respiratory health and increasing the resistance will significantly improve your leg strength. However, it will have very little effect on your arms and upper body strength.

This is the reason why we have strength training in our chart in the previous chapter. On each strength training day, you will work on a different pair of muscle groups. With cycling HIIT, you will burn fats faster. The fat mass in your arms, your gut and your chest will be replaced with muscles giving you a chiseled physique.

To develop a balanced physique, you also need to put some gym time building your upper body strength. In this chapter, we will discuss how you will be able to improve the muscles size and strength in your abdomen, chest, shoulders and upper back. Doing so will also improve the strength in your arms.

The HIIT principle can also be applied to your muscle building routines. To avoid injuries, you must work on different muscle groups every day. By doing this, you will be able to build your muscles in different areas of the body each week. Each muscle group will also have time for repairs before they are used again.

To start your HIIT on building muscles, you need to identify the right weight to use. If you haven't tried using a barbell or a dumbbell in your life, do the following workouts on the various weights suggested. If you could do 10 reps with ease, then you should move on to the next weight level. The objective is to find the best weight where you can consistently do 10 proper repetitions

Type of Exercise	Target Muscle Group	Weight Level 1	Weight Level 2	Weight Level 3	Weight Level 4
Bench Press	Chest	30 pounds	40 pounds	50 pounds	60 pounds
Isolated Dumbbell	Biceps	15 pounds	20 pounds	25 pounds	30 pounds

Curls					
One-arm Triceps Extension	Triceps	10 pounds	15 pounds	20 pounds	30 pounds
Barbell Dead Lift	Back	30 pounds	40 pounds	50 pounds	60 pounds

After finding out the optimum starting weight to use, you need to practice the proper way of execution for each of the exercise movements suggested below. The cheapest way to do this is by looking for exercise videos online. There are a lot of exercise gurus who will show you how to do the exercises properly to avoid injuries. Practice each weight training move before moving on to the HIIT strength program.

Here are the strength training moves that you need to work on:

Seated Isolated Dumbbell Curls

Barbell Squats

One Arm Triceps Extension

Stationary Lunge

Hammer Curls

Triceps Kickback

Bench Press

Bent Over Barbell Row (Wide Grip)

Lying Fly

Incline Dumbbell Bench press

Barbell Dead Lift

Wide Grip Bench Press

Crunches

Leg Raise

Barbell Trunk Rotation

You don't have to learn all of them instantly. You could look them up one by one as the need arises.

Some of these workout moves require a spotter or a partner during working out. You should ask a friend to spot for you if you are working out at home. The gym instructor will usually be the spotter if you are a gym member.

Because you only have 3 workout days left with one rest day, you should work on two muscle groups on each training day. Here are the groups that you need to work on each day:

Day	Pair of Muscle Groups
Tuesday	Arms and Legs
Thursday	Back and Chest
Saturday	Abdominal Muscles and Arms

Most men like having big arms. This is the reason why we work on our arms twice every week. You can replace the arm muscle group with any other muscle group that you want to grow faster and stronger.

Here's the HIIT workout plan that you can follow using the arrangement above:

Day	Workout	Target Muscle Group	Weight	Number of reps	Intensity
Tuesday	Seated Isolated Dumbbell Curls	Biceps	60% of optimum weight	10	High
	Barbell Squats	Legs	optimum weight	10	Low

One Arm Triceps Extension	Triceps	60% of optimum weight	10	High
1-minute Rest				
Stationary Lunge	Legs	Body weight	10	High

	Hammer Curls	Biceps	optimum weight	10	Low
	Triceps Kickback	Triceps	60% of optimum weight	10	High
Thursday	Bench Press	Chest	50% of optimum weigh	10	High

		t		
Bent Over Barbell Row (Wide Grip)	Back	Optimum Weight	10	Low
Lying Fly	Chest	60% of optimum weight	10	High
1				

minute rest				
Incline Dumbbell Bench press	Chest	60% of optimum weight	10	High
Barbell Dead Lift	Back	Optimum Weight	10	Low
Wide Grip	Chest	50% of	10	High

	Bench Press		optimum weight		
Saturday	Crunches	Abdominal Muscles	Body weight	10	High
	Seated Isolated Dumbbell Curls	Biceps	optimum weight	10	Low

Leg Raise	Abdominal Muscles	Body weight	10	High
1-minute rest				
Hammer Curls	Biceps	60% of optimum weight	10	High

Barbell Trunk Rotation	Abdominal Muscles	Optimum Weight	10	Low
Triceps Kickback	Triceps	60% of optimum weight	10	High

To properly execute the HIIT for muscle building, you need to finish the 10 reps of each exercise as fast as you can and move on to the next workout move in the list without resting. As you continue your strength training, the weight will become easier to handle. To keep the workout challenging, you should constantly try out heavier weights.

High intensity weight lifting burns a lot of calories. You will lose a lot of weight if you don't replace the calories that you use up by eating. To build your muscles properly, you need the right combination of carbohydrates and protein. This topic will be discussed later in the book.

Chapter 14: Energy Contribution During 30-Second Sprints

Something unique and beneficial about HIIT workouts is that all the energy pathways described in Lesson 3 are involved. Unlike so many other forms of exercise, HIIT involves both anaerobic and aerobic systems to supply the body with energy. Since there are endless possibilities to structure HIIT workouts, each metabolic pathway will have a different involvement during different HIIT protocols.

The role of each system, the ATP-PC system, the glycolytic system, and the TCA cycle, is to break down and resynthesize ATP, the molecule responsible for energy output in all living things. This is called ATP turnover. The ATP turnover from each energy system depends on a workout's modality, duration, intensity, and volume.

In 1994, Professor Mary Nevill published a study comparing ATP turnover in participants who were repeating two 30-second maximal sprints.11 Here are the results of her study.

ATP turnover in the first sprint:

•ATP-PC system = 21%

•Glycolytic system = 50%

•Aerobic (TCA cycle) = 29%

ATP turnover in the second sprint:

•ATP-PC system = 20%

•Glycolytic system = 36%

•Aerobic (TCA cycle) = 44%

Neville's results show not only that all three energy systems are involved during a

HIIT workout, but that the amount of involvement of each system changes over the course of the workout.

In 2001, Paul Gastin published research showing that aerobic energy system (TCA cycle) contribution can be in the range from 3–69% in a single bout of high intensity exercise, lasting up to 120 seconds. Here is table from that study about energy contribution.12

Duration of Exercise	% Anaerobic Contribution	% Aerobic Contribution
10 seconds	94%	6%
20 seconds	82%	18%
30 seconds	73%	27%
60 seconds	55%	45%
90 seconds	49%	51%

120 seconds	37%	63%

The results in the above table show that as the duration of an exercise bout increases, the contribution from the aerobic system increases as well. But what also happens when the repetitions of HIIT increase is that the ATP turnover from glycolytic system will decrease and the oxidative system will start to take over the ATP resynthesis. When the oxidative system (TCA cycle) becomes the dominant energy provider, it will increase the percentage of type 1 muscle fibers and, therefore, power output will start to decline, something that we'll explore more deeply in the next lesson.

The Big Takeaway

These findings emphasize that the aerobic system (also called oxidative system or TCA cycle) is an important provider to the body's overall energy demand during high intensity interval training. Researchers have concluded that it is work duration, work intensity, and rest duration that affect how quickly aerobic metabolism will start to take over energy contribution in HIIT sessions, which we'll be discussing in the next lesson.

Chapter 15: How To Make The Universe Listen

So I can have anything I want by thinking about it? If this's true, then why are not we all billionaires?

One of the reasons why the law of attraction just fails to work positively on some individuals is that because their vibrations aren't enough to just accomplish their dreams. The failure of the law of attraction to work its wonders is simply often the result of a misalignment of one's conscious & subconscious minds. In order for such a dream to manifest, every single cell of your being must vibrate the exact same frequency. Every part of you must ask the universe just for the exact same thing. Otherwise, there's a conflict within oneself. An internal battle of wills, so to speak. This blurry message confuses the universe which basically tends to answer in kind. Put, if you send the universe a garbled message, then you get a topsy-turvy life.

Take a look at this example:

If you consciously ask for such a promotion but your subconscious brain keeps insisting that the competition is too tough & that you actually won't be promoted, then you're unlikely to get that promotion.

So how do I synchronize my conscious & subconscious minds?

This's done through goal setting, visualization & affirmations. Note that while it's your conscious mind that does the choosing, it's your subconscious that's really responsible for the implementation of the choice. When you just set a goal, you visualize that goal to come true & you affirm it regularly, both the rational & the imaginative sides of your whole brain are actively involved. So what exactly is an affirmation? An affirmation is when you're being in conscious control of your thoughts just by using short, positive, powerful statements to declare. They simply strengthen our beliefs in the potential of an action we just desire to manifest.

Here are some examples of positive affirmations:

" I'm a money magnet, money comes to me easily"

" I'm healthy & happy & i've an amazing relationship with my children"

So, what is the secret on how to meet these goals? Through the habit of using positive affirmations & visualization on a consistent basis to attract what we simply desire.

The subconscious brain is stubborn but it's really possible to reprogram it through affirmations & subliminal messaging which will be just discussed in the succeeding chapters.

I have tried affirmations before. Why did not the universe listen to me then?

Each time you simply think of something, each time you feel something, the universe receives it & reads it. The universe simply considers it as your intention.

First, you really need to clarify your intentions. As previously mentioned, sending mixed signals to the universe will actually get you an ambiguous answer at best. As with writing a letter to such an crucial person, you need to be careful with the wording of your requests. It has to be specific. More importantly, you've to mean it. It should honestly reflect your utmost desires. If it does not sound convincing enough, the universe is likely to reject your request.

If you simply dream of success, then you've to create a face for success. Contemplate on what success means to you. Sort out your goals & prioritize them.

Example:

Do not ask the universe for a soulmate. Tell the universe exactly what you really want for a soulmate. What're his/her defining qualities? What're the things that you've in common? What're the passions that you share? What activities would you do together?

Examples of properly worded intentions are:

I really want a man who cares as much for the environment as I do.

I want a woman who, like me, is passionate about art.

After you have set your intention, then you just need to increase the power of your intention. This may be really done through visualizations, which will be just discussed in detail in the succeeding chapters. Remember that in order for visualizations to work, you really need to see, feel, taste, & hear your goal so vividly in your mind's senses that you can almost see, taste, feel, & hear it with your physical senses.

Next, you need to clear your energy stores. In order for the message to come through, you really need to cleanse the passage through which it'll be transported. What actually clogs up these channels? Negative energy. It finally comes in the form of negative thoughts. That's the fixed mindset voice at the back of your skull whispering: "You really do not deserve it. So you cannot have it." Or "Maybe you deserve it. But because life is unfair, you won't get it."

Clearing your energy stores is all about silencing that strongly embedded voice; thus, just allowing the positive mindset voice to speak up.

Successful ways to just get rid of negative energy include meditation & yoga.

Of course, all these're useless unless you anticipate a response from the universe. When you simply write an email to someone, you expect them to get it. More importantly, you really expect them to answer back. So you check your inbox from time to time. When you order pizza, you just wait for the delivery person to show up in your doorstep. You prepare the exact amount of cash. You might even put a couple of beers in the freezer & just clear the table to make room for the pizza.

You MUST develop the same attitude when sending a request to the universe.

If you asked the universe for a baby, then you really need to anticipate the baby's arrival. Live your lives as though the child is coming soon. This simply means saving enough money for the baby. The future mother needs to eat healthy to just prepare her body for the baby. Take a look at your house. Does it look like there's room for a child? This does not mean you've to buy a bigger home or go crazy shopping for baby clothes, especially if you don't have the money for it. It is the small things that matter like clearing the clutter in your home so it can be kid-friendly. Sometimes, you really need to change your lifestyle. Are you living your life like responsible soon-to-be parents? Maybe it is time to go easy on the drinking. Live your entire life like you are telling the universe: Yes, we are ready for a baby.

Another thing you really need to remember when communicating with the universe is that all the energy you create is useless unless you guide it to the proper direction. You cannot declare it – you really need to take the appropriate ACTIONS towards your goals. For instance, you simply keep asking the universe for a stable relationship with such a great person. But then you keep on dating emotionally unavailable individuals. You keep asking the universe to make you successful. But if you really do not dress for success, then do not expect it to happen. In other words, you really need to live like your dream has already come true. This means making the most out of what the universe has given you.

Lastly, be patient. Recognize that your limited concept of time doesn't apply to the universe. To you, what may actually feel like forever may be nothing but a blink of an eye in other realms. So if your money, your soulmate, or whatever it's that you asked the universe for has not arrived yet, do not give up. Understand that it may take time because environmental conditions need to work & fit together in order to accommodate your wishes.

Instead, you really need to keep your eyes open for opportunities. Sometimes, the universe answers requests in the most unexpected ways. So always just be alert for prospects or else the universe's answer will pass by unnoticed.

If you want your entire life to change, it won't happen if you really keep doing the same old thing that you have been doing for years.

Chapter 16: Combine Hiit With Weight Training For Great Results

If you incorporate weight training into your workout regimen, try adding HIIT or Tabata training sessions to your weight training routines to trim fat and help tone your muscles. I sometimes add a couple Tabata sessions to my workout days and then do full HIIT routines once or twice a week on my days off.

Other times, I incorporate HIIT into my weight training sessions by creating a weight training routine that adds light cardio to intervals of weight lifting. Instead of counting reps during these workouts, I lift for a certain amount of time. Choose weights that will allow you to just barely make it to the end of the interval. It makes for a difficult workout, especially when the lactic acid really starts to build up near the end of the routine.

If you hit a point during an interval where your muscles start to fail, stop just long enough to where you can lift again and get back at it. If you need to, take a 15- to 30-second breather at the end of each interval set.

Here's a template you can use to create your own HIIT weight training routine:

Time/Distance	Exercise	Exertion (1 - 10)
1 minute	Warm up. Light to moderate cardio.	3 to 5
30 seconds	Warm up. Light to moderate	8 to 9

	lifting exercise.	
30 seconds	Heavy lifting exercise. Perform as many lifts as you can in 30 seconds.	8 to 9
15 seconds	Light cardio.	5 to 7

Repeat intervals until 20 minutes have passed.

You could also do the opposite of what's done in the previous workout, opting to do intense cardio during the high-intensity intervals followed by light lifting sessions during the active recovery periods. This is what the alternate workout would look like:

Time/Distance	Exercise	Exertion (1 - 10)
1 minute	Warm up. Light to moderate cardio.	3 to 5
30 seconds	Warm up. Light to moderate lifting exercise.	8 to 9
30 seconds	Intense cardio.	8 to 9
15 seconds	Light lifting exercise.	5 to 7

Repeat intervals until 20 minutes have passed.

The exercises you choose will determine the muscle groups you work in that session. You can opt to concentrate on one muscle group and really hit it hard or you can work different muscle groups to go for a full body routine.

HIIT Tips

The following tips can be used to help ensure you get the most from your workouts while staying safe:

Always warm up. HIIT is intense and can be hard on your body. There's no reason to compound the chance of injury by failing to properly warm up. Light cardio is a good choice for warming up because it gets you moving and begins to elevate your heart rate.

Make sure you choose the right weight. When doing exercises that incorporate weights, choosing the right weight is critical. While you may feel inclined to choose the heaviest weight you can lift, this isn't a good choice because you're going to be doing a lot of reps. You want to choose the heaviest weight you can use to safely perform reps while maintaining good posture. There's a fine line between safe heavy lifting and serious injury. It's up to you to ensure you don't cross it.

Bring it! Push hard during the intense intervals. High-intensity intervals are supposed to be intense. You should be dripping sweat and your heart should be pounding by the time you finish an interval. If not, you probably aren't pushing hard enough.

Make sure you're healthy enough to do HIIT. This type of workout isn't for everyone. If you have health problems, check with your doctor to see if HIIT is a good fit. Even if you don't have health problems, it's a good idea to get a check-up and tell your doctor what you're planning on doing. If you're out of shape, HIIT is going to be extremely tough. There are people who start their fitness journey with HIIT and stick it out, but these people are few and far between. Many beginners would be better served getting in halfway decent shape before trying HIIT.

Keep the intervals short. Most people have a tough time giving everything they've got for 30 seconds. Some athletes can push hard for a minute and elite athletes are able to push for 2 minutes or more. If you're doing intervals that are longer than 2 minutes, you probably aren't doing HIIT. 20-second intervals are the minimum interval length you should be doing.

Mix it up. Don't get stuck on a single workout routine. Your body will get used to doing the same thing over and over and over again. Instead, use different exercise machines and bodyweight workouts to switch things up. Keep your body guessing and you'll be less likely to fall into a rut. You'll also be less likely to burn out and fall victim to repetitive motion injuries.

Don't overdo it. Three HIIT routines a week are all most people should do. Experienced exercisers can push it up to 4 workouts a week. Never do HIIT routines on back-to-back days. Give yourself at least one day between HIIT workouts in order to allow time for your body to recover.

Listen to your body. HIIT sessions are intense. They can take a toll on your body, especially when combined with other types of exercise and/or lifting. If you're extremely sore or have a nagging pain that just won't go away, it may be a good idea to forget about HIIT until your body has had a chance to heal. You don't want to suffer an injury that'll sideline you for weeks or even months. Most injuries come about as a result of people ignoring early indicators that there's a problem. Small problems can become large problems in a hurry if they're ignored.

Chapter 17: Applying Hiit To Calisthenics

You can apply HIIT even when using bodyweight exercises. Using HIIT with calisthenics workouts will improve your muscular and aerobic conditioning at the same time. There are hundreds of calisthenics workouts out there. You should pick the ones that you can do effectively.

This chapter will show some examples of HIIT protocols using calisthenics workouts. You may replace some of the calisthenics exercises suggested in this chapter according to your preferred intensity level. You may refer to the section below that suggests alternatives for the suggested workout moves.

General Calisthenics HIIT Routine

High Intensity: Jumping Jacks – Do it fast for 1 minute

Plank – Try to keep the position and your abdominal muscles tight for 30 seconds

High Intensity: Burpees – Do as many as you can in one minute

Alternative Lunges – Do as many as you can in one minute but make sure that you keep the correct form

High Intensity: Mountain Climber – Do a high-intensity round for 30 seconds

Pushups – Do slow pushups for 1 minute

You should take a two-minute break after each round. You should do the routine 3-6 times in a session depending on the amount of time you have available.

Alternative workouts

If for some reason, you cannot do any of the high intensity calisthenics exercises, you can replace them with the following workouts:

- Spiderman pushups

- Shadow boxing

- Squats

- Leg flutter

- Bicycles

You can replace the workouts that you cannot execute properly. You should do as many reps as you can in the given time for these high-intensity workouts, however, you should make sure that you do the correct form.

This is a general routine that is designed to workout your whole body. If you are planning to isolate certain muscle groups, you can replace the suggested workouts with ones that work on your target muscle groups.

If you want to focus on your core muscles for a particular day for example, you can do this routine instead:

High Intensity: Bird Dog Crunch (1 minute)

Plank (30 Seconds)

High Intensity: Planks with knee bends (1 minute)

L-Sit (30 Seconds)

High Intensity: Burpees (1 minute)

Crunches (1 minute)

Do the routine 3-6 times.

As you can see, all the workouts in this routine area focused on the core. Only burpees are a multi-joint workout move. By doing this workout, you will be able to put a lot of stress in your abs and your back muscles using solely bodyweight exercises.

You can do your own HIIT calisthenics routine for other muscles groups. Because you are using your bodyweight in calisthenics workouts, you cannot isolate specific muscles like the biceps and the triceps. Instead, you are only targeting multiple muscles groups with multi-joint exercises. Common workout moves, like pushups for example, use not only your arms but also you back and your chest. You will also need help from your core to keep your body straight while you are doing it.

Upper Body HIIT Calisthenics Routine

Here is an example of a routine that focuses on improving your upper body strength:

High Intensity: Pushups (1 minute)

Triceps dip (1 minute)

High Intensity: Chin-ups (1 minute)

Decline pushups (1 minute)

High Intensity: Pull ups (30 Seconds)

Flexed-arm hang (30 seconds)

Doing 3-6 sets of this routine will work out your back, chest and arm muscles. Your entire upper body will benefit from these types of HIIT routines.

You can also apply HIIT principles to your lower body muscles. This includes all your large muscles from the waist down.

Lower Body HIIT Calisthenics Routine

High Intensity: Step ups   (1 minute)

Wall sit (1 minute)

High Intensity: Squats (1 minute)

Walking lunges (30 seconds)

High Intensity: Jump on box (1 Minute)

Reverse lunges (30 Seconds)

Just like with all the other previously suggested routines, most beginners will be able to do these calisthenics workouts. If you are just doing your HIIT at home with no past workout experience, these calisthenics exercises will be the best workouts to start with.

If you have access to free weights, you may also use them to increase the intensity of your workouts.

Chapter 18: Using Resistance Training With Hiit

As you become better in executing calisthenics exercises, you will notice that you no longer become easily exhausted by bodyweight training. Your body will be lighter by the end of the second week.

If you have access to free weights and resistance elastics, you should use them to make the workouts more challenging. By using free weights, you will be able to increase the intensity of common calisthenics exercises.

If doing bodyweight squats is no longer exhausting for example, you can carry a 20 lbs. dumbbell or kettlebell while doing it. This will slow you down in your execution. It will make the workout more challenging and you will become easily exhausted even when doing workouts that you are familiar with.

In the beginning, you should simply add weights to some of your favorite calisthenics exercises. As you progress however, you need to do routines with workouts that target specific muscles. Some of these workouts cannot be done with without weights or resistance.

Chest HIIT Routine with free weights

Instead of targeting your entire upper body, you can make a routine that will work on the specific muscles you want to develop. Here is an example of a routine that you can use to improve your chest muscles:

High Intensity: Butterfly press (1 minute)

Pushups (1 minute)

High Intensity: Bench press (1 minute)

Decline pushups (1 minute)

High Intensity: Pull ups (30 Seconds)

Flexed-arm hang (30 seconds)

When doing high intensity weighted workouts, you need to make sure that you work with weights a few pounds below your maximum weight limit. If you work with your maximum, you will not be able to push yourself to do many reps in the given time. If you do your reps fast with your maximum weight, you may become injured or you may let go of the weights.

You should also make sure that you have a spotter when doing dangerous moves like the bench press.

Resistance tools to use for beginners

Use Dumbbells

If you are planning to purchase equipment for doing HIIT, you should choose to buy dumbbells. Dumbbells are easy to use and they make common workout moves more difficult. If you are confident in doing lunges for example, you will find it more challenging if you do it with a dumbbell in each hand. Most of the workouts that you can do with barbells can also be done with dumbbells. With just a pair, you will be able to do a wide range of exercises.

Resistance elastics

You can also use resistance bands or tubes to make your workouts more intense. They are easier to store than dumbbells but they can be a good alternative to their heavier counterpart. You can also do most of the weight exercises with them. By attaching the band to the floor for example, you will be able to pull the band upwards using motions similar to doing curls.

Chapter 19: Common Mistakes

When Doing Hiit

HIIT is, beyond doubt, a very effective workout but to get results, it needs to be done correctly. Most people are not used to pushing themselves as hard as necessary for HIIT especially for a workout that is as short as 7- 10 minutes because it is extremely uncomfortable.

That is why many people often start making mistakes during their workouts which can easily sabotage their efforts and diminish their results. Here is a look at some of the most common mistakes to avoid when doing HIIT.

Opting For Longer Workouts

Essentially, a HIIT session can last anywhere from four to twenty minutes, or thirty minutes if stretched to the maximum. If someone is able to push it beyond that, then that is not an achievement.

It is a common error to go for longer sessions during HIIT. The whole point is to push your body to the maximum limit during high intensity periods. This will automatically make your sessions shorter as the body will be too exhausted to work anymore.

Not Warming Up

HIIT training can be tough and strenuous, especially for beginners who are not yet ready to use their body's maximum potential during their workout sessions. Even those who are physically fit and active need to warm up before they start with their HIIT training.

It is a common mistake to directly hit the gym and get going with the session. This will reduce the effects that you are trying to achieve. Without a warm up, the body will not be able to give it's all during the high intensity intervals.

Choosing Complex And Complicated Movements

Experts say that with subsequent sessions of workouts, the body can get too tired to perform a complex movement. During your first session, a complicated movement might not seem that bad at all. But after repeated movements, the body and brain could be overstrained, increasing the chances of an injury such as sprains or falls.

Instead, it is advised to choose movements for HIIT workouts that are easier to perform, without having to put too much thought into which body part goes where and which muscle to stretch more than the other.

Apart from choosing complex movements, another common mistake is not perform the easy ones correctly. As simple as a movement might be, unless you are performing it right, it is not going to be effective.

It is always good to give your mind and body a chance to master a movement first before you start training faster.

Not Paying Attention To 'Recovery' Intervals

This is one of the most common mistakes during HIIT to reduce the resting or recovery intervals in an attempt to make it 'tougher'. This is the wrong idea.

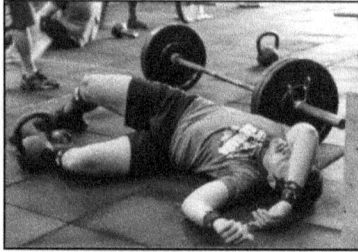

The recovery period is as important as the high intensity interval, if not more. This is the period where the muscles pay off what is called an 'oxygen debt'. They receive the oxygen that they were deprived off as the workout proceeded and led up to their fatigue. Once they get the oxygen back, they can work just as hard in the next high intensity period. If ample recovery time is not taken, then muscles are only partially ready for the next hard work.

Not Being 'Intense' Enough

By high intensity during HIIT training, it is meant that you should be extremely breathless, the heart thumping loudly against your chest and your body and brain both screaming that you cannot push any further. If this does not happen to you during your high intensity intervals, you are making the same mistake as many others: not going hard enough.

You need to push yourself to the point where you physically and mentally reach a point beyond which you know you cannot go on. Only then will your HIIT workout be a success.

Most HIIT training sessions involve movements and exercises that are natural and easy. They make the workout more effective and also reduce the chances of an injury. Lifting weights can also be a part of high interval sessions but these weights should not be too heavy. The easier they are to lift, the better.

Diet And Clothing Matter

As good as it might look, wearing clothes that are too tight are only going to bother you during the workout. It is important to invest in proper gym clothes that are made of a breathable material, do not trap sweat against your skin and leave you itchy. It is also necessary to wear proper trainers for your sessions.

In terms of nutrition, first and foremost is to stay hydrated! Drink ample water well before your workout session starts because it's about to get sweaty!

There are many protein shakes available, which can be used. Otherwise a good fibre and lean protein meal works just as fine. Having said that, it is best to be done eating at least an hour before your session. It is a common error to eat right before working out and not pay attention to what you eat either. Fruits and vegetables just before working out are not going to be very helpful.

Not Staying Determined Enough

The last thing your body needs to hear is 'You can't do it!' Yet it hears this a lot during HIIT training. HIIT can be very tough and demanding. It can make the body feel more exhausted than ever. So it is common to give up. It will feel hard and impossible, and the negative thinking will only make it worse. But sticking to it will allow you to reap some great benefits.

Doing HIIT Too Often

Boasted by the great outcome and result of HIIT training can lead to the mistake of over doing it such as, trying to do it every day. This is not good for the muscles at all. The maximum frequency of a HIIT session should not be more than twice or thrice a week. This is to allow ample recovery time to the body so that it is all set for the next round.

This is primarily why many people have begun to prefer this over long everyday sessions of low intensity workouts. It does not demand too much time from their busy routines.

Choosing The Wrong Timing

Randomly choosing half an hour in the week for HIIT workout is a big mistake. The sessions need to be timed properly. Having a session right after you eat or just before bed is a bad idea.

In fact, the sooner in the day you train, the better. Taking a good but light breakfast early in the morning, an hour before the HIIT session is the best way to go about it. This way your fat reserves will be targeted better. It will also prepare your body to burn the calories you will be munching up throughout the day.

As a matter of fact, working out early and before going to work will also maximize your performance there, as the concentration and productivity will be at its best.

Chapter 20: More About Tabata Hiit

Tabata is a style of HIIT that has been proven by research to build up your endurance and your strength in the shortest time possible. This is because it consists of sessions of total effort, repeated, with short rest periods. Here's how you can bring Tabata HIIT into your regular workout.

Choose your exercise

Choose from these:

Box jumps

Burpees

Jumping lunges

Mountain climbers

Squat into overhead presses

Use this formula:

20 seconds of high intensity activity with your chosen exercise

Rest for 10 seconds

Repeat 7 more times

Rest for one minute

Choose another exercise:

Choose another and repeat the above or you could give yourself a large pat on the back for one of the hardest exercise regimes you have ever done – in just four minutes.

When you think it's time to make that healthy change, Tabata is the kick-ass calorie burner you are looking for and, if you add in some strength training as well, there really is no limit to your potential achievements. This next training example is a real energy busting routine and if you can complete it successfully, you will be ready to take on the world!

Here it is:

Equipment

You will need a timer and a set of dumbbells

Tabata – each exercise is done alternately for 20 seconds work, 10 seconds rest for four minutes total

Strength – each exercise is done alternately for 30 seconds work until you have completed 3 reps of each one

Tabata – each exercise is done alternately for 20 seconds work, 10 seconds rest for four minutes total

Conclusion

With a little training and practice, you can quickly achieve massive results from HIIT. Don't neglect this powerful type of training that can be adapted to a large variety of workouts.

Let's stay in touch! You can pick up a free guide to Tabata training and some additional tips to keep you on track, here: